MARROW ME:

One Man's Entrance into the Merry World of Multiple Myeloma

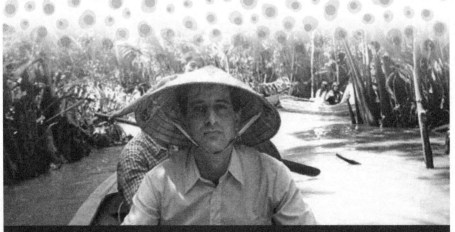

A MEMOIR BY JOSHUA ROBERTS

Marrow Me

Joshua Roberts

with comments and afterword by his sisters

BITINGDUCK PRESS
ALTADENA, CA

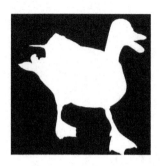

Published by Bitingduck Press
ISBN 978-1-938463-73-0
© 2019 Margot Roberts Sweed
For information contact
Bitingduck Press, LLC
Altadena, California
notifications@bitingduckpress.com
http://www.bitingduckpress.com
Cover art by Ross Sweed

Publisher's Cataloging-in-Publication
Roberts, Joshua [1961-2017   ]

Marrow Me/by Joshua Roberts–1st ed.—Altadena, CA: Bitingduck
Press, 2019
p. cm.

Contents—personal account of battle with multiple myeloma.

[1. Memoir –Nonfiction 2. Cancer—Treatment—Complications and
Sequelae—Failure. 3.Plasma Cell Diseases—multiple myeloma] I. Title

ISBN 9781938463730
LCCN 2019943200

For A., my country priest

I am a Figure of Fun

– Nick Cave

I wish I knew a prayer that wasn't me, me, me. Help *me*. Let *me* be happier. Let *me* die soon. Me, me, me.

—*The End of the Affair*, Graham Greene

I stood in the disenchanted field
Amid the stubble and the stones,
Amazed, while a small worm lisped at me
The song of my marrow-bones.

—"End of Summer," Stanley Kunitz

Chapter One

CONTENTS

"WHAT HAVE YOU GOT IN this thing?"

Mock-grumbled by Miriam, an assistant at the public health school for which we both work, as she staggers alongside me down the early-evening sidewalk lugging my overnight bag. It's a scuffed black bag I'm unable to carry even the three measly blocks to Suburban Station.

Miriam is good-natured to be sure; she is exaggeratedly complaining for my amusement as well as her own. I *think*.

She is funny, much younger than me, black clothes and variously dyed hair, a recommender of good books, her cubicle adorned with pictures of Nick Cave, Johnny Cash, Robert Mitchum in the original *Cape Fear*. She is considerate and her fiancé is fortunate. When my spine compacted the previous week in the lobby of the school building, she ran to get me the number of her chiropractor, made sure I got through on my cell phone for an emergency appointment, saw me into a cab to his office.

Not that any of that did me a bit of good, not with what it turns out I really have, but, you know—it's the thought, as is often said, that counts. Now here is Miriam once again, volunteering to carry my bag for me so I won't miss my train. Ensuring she'll only have to work this much later, or at any rate *harder*, when she returns to the office to finish her assignments before she can clear off her desk and head out for home and resume her private life.

Grumble, grumble. It's okay, Miriam, you can be pissed for real, it's all right.

Me, I am barely managing to carry two envelopes. Okay, not any ordinary envelopes: twin jumbo packets from Thomas Jefferson University Hospital, too wide and unfoldable for my bag, containing my x-ray and MRI films. These are of some importance, since I'm on my way from downtown Philadelphia to Bucks County to spend the night with my older sister Margot and her family before being admitted first thing next morning to the Fox Chase Cancer Center (FCCC). The doctors there will need to see the films.

If not for my sister, a nurse practitioner at FCCC who leapt into action the instant I phoned with my results, who leap-frogged me over hurdles to get an immediate appointment with a leading specialist, I don't know what I'd be doing at this moment. Weeping in the gutter is a good possibility. Like I said, I can't even carry my overnight bag. I've got at least two vertebral fractures in my lower spine that the OxyContin I've begun taking (40+ milligrams daily, in 12-hour time-re-lease capsules) has not quite managed to make me forget. The films under my arm are proof of that, or so a couple of doctors have already informed me.

I haven't been able to make myself examine those images close-ly yet: my own personal Halloween in the x-rays, or even worse, the cross-sections of the MRI, organs and tissues and cavities laid out in magnetic slices like so much blue-tinted barbecue. But I feel their infor-mation with every careful step: my skeleton is crumbling, frangible as crackers. Dunk my skull in your soup and watch it dissolve.

What have I got in that thing? Open up the bag, Miriam, see for yourself, dump it out on the sidewalk. I'm so doped up I can't re-member what-all I threw in there. The nervous junk of a newly-mint-ed cancer patient, I expect: toilet kit, shoes, underwear and socks, a growing folder of medical records, rattling bottles of various painkillers (Where are you now, oh little white bottle of Motrin®? You were the very first medication I bought to deal with my growing back pain. Sad little over-the-counter bottle. But it wasn't your fault! You did your best! You didn't know it was cancer! *Je vous salue, petite bouteille blanche de*

Motrin®.), holiday presents for my sister's two boys, some books and magazines that the meds and my steady low-grade panic won't let me focus on anyway.

Four days before, I was officially diagnosed with multiple myeloma, a "treatable" but essentially incurable form of blood cancer, very rare in 44-year-old males such as me. I've never smoked, have exercised regularly since youth (hiking, swimming, biking), have kept alcohol intake to moderate levels since my mid-20s and am a near-vegetarian. I'm not sure what type of overnight packing is required to deal with the Cosmic Carcinoma Crotch-kick.

My boss, the dean of the school—of whom I have always been politely terrified—met with me an hour ago to discuss the likely terms of my absence from the school, the possibilities of working from home or hospital as treatments begin. She gave me her home and cell phone numbers (this is major), assured me that treatments for myeloma patients improve yearly (she's an M.D.), with many productive clinical trials currently in effect and even more on the horizon. People live long and active lives with this type of cancer, she told me.

And then, before I left her office, Dean G. did something which before this day would have been inconceivable to either of us, or certainly to me. She rose from behind her desk to hug me very carefully as any dear relative would, and I knew she meant it deeply.

I'm doomed.

It is Monday, December 19, 2005, passing 4:30 PM. The yellow discs of the City Hall tower clock assume power in the falling dusk. William Penn's statue considers us all. The streets and sidewalks are beginning to clog. Don't bump into me, please. I walk like a frightened robot, not daring to pivot at the waist. At Suburban Station on 16th Street, I follow Miriam and my bag down the gritty stairs, holding to the banister all the way, then shuffle off to buy my one-way ticket.

Miriam is determined to see me off and comes further underground with me to the train platform, waiting with me for the West Trenton local, setting the bag at my feet with a last mimed flourish of Herculean effort. Ho ho, kiddo: believe me when I say my sides are splitting. I make sure to stand against a platform pillar, my back to the painted concrete, so no one can jostle me from behind. If I happen to trip,

I'll yell at anyone who tries to lift me, convinced the helping hands of strangers will only snap something else.

The train arrives with its rubber stink and hiss of brakes. Not especially late, either, a tribute to the fine minds who run the Southeastern Pennsylvania Transportation Authority.

"Good luck, Josh!" Miriam waves. Did she kiss my cheek? I can't remember everything clearly. (You'll be hearing *that* from me again). But her look of concern remains clear in my mind. Goodbye, Miriam! Thanks! I can take it from here!

I kick my bag across the platform and onto the train, after the other commuters have already boarded. I keep kick-shoving it down the aisle of the car till I find an empty window seat. I lay the film envelopes across my lap, my ticket out for the conductor, my other hand death gripping the armrest as we start to move. We're still underground, but after a few minutes of lurching rumble the train emerges into the open wastes of North Philadelphia and I see that night has come.

Rising into the dark in the illuminated car, my head is reflected in the scratched window, riding over the tired bricks and wires of the passing city, and I watch the expression on my face, my skin, the wrapping, the envelope, the outmost layer of the bag of me. Ok, tough guy, what are you made of? What have you got in this thing?

Chapter Two

SHOW ME

OW THIS IS JUST THE sort of thing I'd hoped to avoid, and
here I am doing it right at the start, in the opening pages of
the story: describing myself contemplating myself. Me reflecting upon
my reflection. *Me* looking at *me*. Me *writing* about me. **ME** and **MY**
MEmoir of **MY** Multipl**E** **MY**eloma. Me, me, me. This is just the sort
of thing I'd hoped to avoid forever.

By way of example: "Suicide? That's the last thing you should do,"
cracks The Devil in the excellent film comedy *Bedazzled* (I mean the
British original, of course, not the bogus Hollywood remake), and The
Prince of Darkness might as well have been speaking of memoirs, too.
They're supposed to be how you *finish*. Writing one of those was never
part of the plan, was not, literarily speaking, how I expected to introduce myself to the world. *Marrow Me?* Are you kidding?

Once that train leaves the station, what's to stop me from going the
full route with a whole *series* of memoirs, milking my disease for all
its tragicomically worth? Can we expect the transgressive, brooding
yet shockingly hilarious cancer sequels: *Myeloma Nation, Running with
Stem Cells, A Bone Breaking Work of Just Plain Staggering, The Osteoblast Veil*
(always good for a laugh at hematology seminars) and, my personal
favorite— 12 weeks on the *USA Today* bestseller list, soon to be a major
pirated download—*Heave, Splay, Lose.*

If at any time before my diagnosis I *had* considered a memoir, some
sort of personal narrative intended for the general reading public, I

imagined it appearing only towards the end of a long life and respectable career, sometime in my 70s or 80s (or even my 100s, no need to rush things), when I might conceivably have something worthwhile to say about the world after several decades of poking around in it, something to say that wasn't simply all *me*. I'll confess to having picked a title for *that* imaginary book some time ago: *Self-Loathing*. You like it? Well, I don't. I *hate* it. *I* hate it because *I* picked it. I hate *me*.

Sociological digression: Christopher Lasch published *The Culture of Narcissism* in 1979, and if anything, his book now seems touchingly quaint in its anticipation of where we're at today, our early-21st-century and counting. *The Culture of Narcissism* is subtler than its famous title suggests: it is not the simple condemnation of egomania it's often taken for, but instead a layered portrayal of the condition of chronic self-absorption without productive self-improvement, the incapability of truly understanding one's own flaws, the permanent inability to correct those flaws in any effective manner. True narcissism (Lasch argued) is not self-love but rather something with roots in the opposite end of the emotional spectrum: deep insecurity; the conviction that one is not attractive enough, rich enough, famous enough for the artificial standards by which our culture judges success; a neurotic obsession with personal disappointment, combined with the constant worry that others see us as disappointing; a terminal *neediness*; a failure to obtain satisfaction or even basic happiness from one's real self. And our culture (Western consumer culture, Society-of-the-Spectacle culture, yes, I'm looking at *you*) has only evolved to stroke and feed and promote this condition to more stupefying levels since Lasch described it in 1979. Our flaws are no longer meant to be fixed, they are instead to be *nurtured*. More: they are expected to be *broadcast*, properly *aired*, made commercially viable.

This is what "advances" in technology and communication have brought us to: Facebook, Myspace, YouTube, Twitter, Thisser, Thatter, Whateverer—every computer and smartphone a vanity press, hosting ever-swelling armies of self-publishing selves, cranking out blog posts and tweets and uploading their terribly interesting personal videos and sometimes even producing actual printed books, the emphasis never on "I have a tale to tell" but always on "*I* have a tale to tell...and guess what, it's all about *me!* Look what happened to me, listen to what I have to say about what I watched on TV last night and how my parents were mean to me when I was five years old. Look at how many friends I have, hundreds of them, thousands of them, you can tell they're my friends because they clicked the "Like" button on my profile. By the way, have I told you how much I drank last night, because I really do drink quite a lot, and snort too much, too, and my childhood was too much and...wait, where are you going? Don't listen to *her*, listen to *me! me! me!* Put *me* on TV, make a movie out of *my* blog, everyone stop what they're doing and pay attention to *my* hurt feelings, *my* scraped knee, if you stop paying attention to my endless screech for attention I will so totally die!"

From Milan Kundera's *The Book of Laughter and Forgetting* (1978): "Once the writer in every individual comes to life (and that time is not far off) we are in for an age of universal deafness and lack of understanding." Consider the outrageous elitism of that statement, the frightening whiff of self-hatred in that statement, the undeniable *truth* of that statement.

But enough of me talking about how much I hate people who talk about themselves. What do *you* think about me talking about how much I hate people who talk about themselves? Because I'm no better than anyone else involved in this racket. Of *course*, I am here to presume upon your time, with my precious sob story of how I have spent the past years suffering from my particular disease, my gingerbread bones, my mutant blood, boo hoo, poor widdle me. I am dancing for your pennies as shamelessly as anyone and no use pretending I'm not. Notice me, notice me, step right up! See The Boy with the Cureless Cancer! One swipe of one thin credit card allows you in! See the Protein Kid with the Question-Mark Spine! Alive, alive, alive...but for how much longer? Order now before it's too late!

What else did you *think* I was doing? Oh, the shame. I was hoping to publish at least one book before I croaked, I just didn't plan for it to be about the croaking process itself. So much for the mask of art (well, maybe not "art"; let's just call it "made-up stuff") that I'd hoped to hide behind. My life's goal has always been to hide my life. And boy, am I off to a fine start. Reader, prepare yourself for the worst...

THE EMBARRASSING SECTION THAT MUST BE DISPENSED WITH AS EXPEDITIOUSLY AS POSSIBLE

As stated, a memoir was bottom-most on my list of things to do in life. There was all this other writing of mine that was supposed to make a different sort of impression, possibly even becoming a career of sorts, beginning in college when I first attempted serious literary production, intent on novels, stories, *fiction*, objective literary *fiction* in which I would not figure very much at all. Nobody was supposed to learn about *me*. "Reveal nothing personal" was my motto, or, better still, "Reveal nothing personal, not even *that*."

Flaubert, Joyce, Nabokov were my models (might as well aim high, I figured): the cold steel pen, the silence, the exile, the cunning, all that high Olympian detachment. That was what I felt, and still feel, the best literature to be. Not the writer's dishwater life but the sentences he or she turns out, the chapters and characters and finished works set down in sweaty effort, line by effortful line: *they* were the point of the daily struggle at the desk, to which the breathing/feeding/defecating organism behind them functions merely as an adjunct.

So, okay, fiction: there's been some. I've managed to get some stories published, beginning with a couple of efforts in very small chapbooks right after college, and a few more in slightly-larger-circulation journals in the 1990s, and I attended some of the better writing conferences (Bread Loaf, Sewanee) whereat I received some much-appreciated head-pats, and in 2005 I even placed a story in a well-regarded journal whose contributors have included Nobel Prize winners. Not that I'm bragging or anything. Who, *me?* You must have me confused with some *other* asshole memoirist. I just want the record to show that this fiction-writing dream of mine was not completely delusional, that I really did get published and paid for my trouble once in a very great while.

But no books, no novels, nope-sirree—not in print, anyway. There were supposed to be novels, there *had* to be novels, that's where the action is. (Or *was*. Now it's in memoirs, seems like). And there *were* novels, two and a half of them and one novella, now collecting dust in basement cartons and other spider holes around my house. Let me tell you about the last of these, titled *Mars* (which ain't science fiction, but takes place here on Earth, with regular people and everything). Worked on it from 1998 through the beginning of 2001 while holding down a full-time job, scribbling and typing every weekday before dawn and most of every Sunday, too. I was in my late 30s by then and figured if I didn't get it right this time, I never would. I rewrote and rewrote the first chapters, obsessed with "the perfect opening," one that would snare the reader straight away and never give him or her a chance to put the book down or think of anything else. I began to contact agents, some of whom I had already met at those conferences, or to whom I'd been referred by some of the chummier writers I knew, and one after another those agents politely turned the manuscript aside. But that was okay. There were loads of agents around. I wasn't going to let one or three or fifteen rejections halt my juggernaut. Somewhere out there (preferably in New York City, but *somewhere*) there had to be a hungry agent starting out, some operator who'd want to take a chance...

Finally, in the spring of 2001, I found one. He was a junior agent without much experience, but the agency he worked for was major. One of my favorite authors was a client of theirs. This, I'd been told, was the best possible situation to be in: representation by an eager young starter at an established firm, someone willing to take risks in a way the head agent might not, and with the reputation of his agency to back him up. I yipped, I danced. A big-time agency in New York City wanted to go to bat for my novel! I couldn't believe my luck.

And I *shouldn't* have. The agent couldn't sell the fucking thing. All he managed to do was prove right all the other agents who'd turned it down: no publisher wanted to invest their money in *Mars*, even if they thought it was any good. Editors who read the novel didn't seem to think it was badly written, only that it was too much of a marketing challenge:

"...I'm sorry to report that we don't believe [we] could publish this project successfully for the author, even though it tempted us."

And:

"[A] book like this depends on sharing the same sense of humor. I have always maintained that mine is oblique, odd, and not shared by many people on the planet. That, unfortunately, leads me to not quite getting books like Mars."

And:

"Thank you so much for sending Mars...I spent far too much time with this novel, I'm afraid, mostly because [the] writing is terrific and even though this isn't the type of novel I usually go for, I kept thinking about it...But the truth is, it's got a little too much darkness...and ultimately the grimness of the book left me cold. I couldn't fix on any one character to love, and with me it has to be love...."

Dark, grim, no one to love: I fail to see the problem here. Who wouldn't want to settle down on the couch with a sweet read like that? With its hydra-headed storylines and bee-colony of characters, like the real-estate mogul driven mad by the idea that there is gold ore beneath the foundation of his signature office tower in downtown Philadelphia; the MFA student exploiting his girlfriend by concocting a memoir (Yes! A pox on memoirs!) about their sex life with text cut-and-pasted from porno chatrooms; the edible board game; the neo-Unabomber figure; the prize goose whose sawed-off beak makes a necklace for a serial rapist. And that's just for starters. I tried to make it funny. That was always the main idea, that Mars would be comical, that it would make readers laugh, except of course for when it was making them sick to their stomachs.

Here's how one agent, back when I was still trawling for one, took the trouble to break it down for me over the phone:

"I would love to sell something of yours. This manuscript you've sent me has a lot of good writing. But the thing is, your book is just too complicated, and publishers today don't want anything that's the least bit complicated. I can't imagine anyone who would try and sell such a thing."

"But what am I supposed to do? Cut storylines? Cut characters? They're all connected to each other."

"No. Just write another book. Start again, write something new, make it simple and uncomplicated. Write something direct and get back to me then. Write something from your bones."

Okay, I made that last line up, but that's essentially what the man said. Even then, I appreciated the time he took to phone me and offer a sort of encouragement. In many ways that fellow was more supportive than the guy who actually was my agent. Because this guy, late in 2002, e-mailed to tell me he was leaving the publishing world. I don't believe he was more than 25 years old, but it just wasn't for him, you see. In a final attempt to ease the sting, he closed by stating that he'd gone into "the book biz" in order to get novels like mine into print and he was sorry he hadn't been able to make that happen.

I'm not sure that he ever managed to place anybody's manuscript anywhere.

My attempts to secure representation elsewhere, either at my original agency or others, got no place fast. Naturally I had to tell prospective agents where *Mars* had been, naturally they were none too thrilled to learn its submission history, naturally the manuscript never left my hard drive or the basement.

While all that was going on, I had started another novel. You people want uncomplicated, I'll give you uncomplicated! Here was the simple, uncomplicated idea I had for my next smash work: a novel about five computer programmers laboring within a top-secret military-industrial compound in the Nevada desert in 1966, shot through with tones of Philip K. Dick-style hallucinatory paranoia and Cold War terror, with elaborate detours into the general history and evolution of computer programming language. What could be simpler? I completed perhaps 100 pages of draft before shelving the damn thing for good. (It was too complicated!) For the record, a boiled-down extract of this attempt appeared as a story, "Revolver," in issue #61 of *AGNI* (Spring 2005), just in time for my 44th birthday.

So that was it. I gave up. I'm no novelist, no fiction writer, not these days at any rate. I can only think of the true writers, slogging away at their desks every day no matter what the world throws at them. *Especially* in the face of what the world throws at them.

I think of the magnificent Stanley Elkin, one of the criminally underappreciated greats, who produced books regularly from 1964 until his death in 1995, despite miserable health (multiple sclerosis diagnosed at age 42, in combination with severe heart problems) and the stunning indifference of the reading public. He never let his poor sales and worse body halt or even slow his output; I cannot praise enough the majesty of his novels *The Dick Gibson Show*, *Searches and Seizures*, or *The Rabbi of Lud*, to name just three of his outstanding books, all howlingly funny and deeply sad and brilliantly stylish. *That* was a writer. I can't do *that*. I look in my bag (this is my "bag of writer's tricks" I'm talking about now) and ask: what have I got in this thing? *Nothing much* is the answer, it seems, and I don't particularly care any more.

In the meantime, I settled into the routines of the work-a-day, and I can't say I have much to complain about there. After too many years of low-paid gray-collar office work meant only to keep a rented roof over my head and basic food on my thrift-store table until such time as the world came to recognize my stupendous literary gifts (I'll wait until you finish laughing), I knuckled down and got a Master's degree in what is now called *Information* (as opposed to *Library*) Science, which eventually led to a fairly decent position: librarian and webmeister and general IT guy at a public health school in Philadelphia, within the same university where I got my M.S. I know how very fortunate I am to be here. Ten years now and counting, with health coverage and a pension plan, and I've paid off my grad-school loans. When I happen to be reminded of my days (my fanatical-termite, Simon-the-Stylite days) as a writer, I consider them fully over.

Except that now a topic worth writing about has dropped into my lap.

THIS CONCLUDES THE MOST EMBARRASSING SECTION

*B*ECAUSE IT'S HARDLY MY OWN topic, is it? Neither myeloma nor cancer generally. This is not exactly some unique case we're talking about. "I only am escaped alone to tell thee," as a succession of survivors are said to have told Job? No: not only because I *haven't* escaped, but because I'm hardly alone, not by the longest of shots. There are approximately 20,000 new cases of myeloma diagnosed each year just in the United States, where more than 100,000 patients are presently seeking treatment. The disease remains incurable and too-little-known to the public.

Worst of all, while the American Cancer Society reports that cancer rates are, happily, in a general decline, those relating to myeloma are on the rise, with the disease appearing in ever-younger patients. There has been a tremendous broadening of interest in this disease in the past decade and a half, especially within the medical and pharmaceutical industries, which recognize wide-open territory when they see it. New treatments are yielding positive results, extending life expectancies.

Myeloma patients and activists have been profiled in national magazines and on network morning shows. Kathy Giusti, founder of the Multiple Myeloma Research Foundation, has received numerous awards for leadership, including being named one of *Time* magazine's 100 most influential people in the world and an Open Science Champion of Change by President Obama. Some famous people have died from it: Actors Peter Boyle and Roy Scheider, and former NFL linebacker Elijah Alexander, founder of the Tackle Myeloma Foundation. The fact was not kept out of their obituaries.

So myeloma awareness is being raised to a degree, and I mean here to do my part to raise it a bit higher. I repeat: while I intend to crack jokes like myeloma cracks bones, this is a deadly serious disease, and even while its treatment has vastly improved, there is nothing like a cure at the moment. There are too many people staring at their faces in the dirty train window, scared of where the train is taking them, terrified of their own reflection in the nighttime glass. I'm not convinced that *my* story needs to be told, but I know that the story of myeloma patients, and the efforts to contain and eradicate their disease, must be, so I'm coming at this thing with the only tools I have, the ones at the ends of each arm, my own two typing hands: dry skin and chancy bone and muddled blood. *They're* what I've got in this thing, and I might as well put them at the service of others.

Let me tell you a story about someone else:

The Wednesday before Thanksgiving, 2007. Thanksgiving Eve: one of my favorite interludes of the year. In keeping with tradition, work had let out early, which is how I pulled up on my bike outside the neighborhood supermarket just before three in the afternoon, dismounting, doffing my helmet. Slightly less than a year before, the oncologist who oversaw my stem-cell transplant at the Hospital of the University of Pennsylvania declared my myeloma officially in remission, and I am scooting around the city as of old, cycling like nobody's business, a loaded pack on my back bothering me not at all.

Someone called my name. From across the street, a woman called my name out of the open door of a beauty salon, and she approached me in a hurry, mortifyingly unrecognizable—short blond hair, black leotard and sweater—calling my name, waving and smiling.

Godammit, who the hell is it?

Thank goodness she says her name: "It's me, Lainie." And I had a bit of an alibi for not recognizing her: we hadn't seen each other for years, since back when her hair was black and down over her shoulders.

But still, *she* pegged *me* from across the street. Another reminder of how most people have far better social skills than I do.

Lainie and I had worked together in a miserable court-reporting agency in the early 1990s, where I was a proofreader and she a reporter. One of the few pleasant memories I had of that place involved seeing her get together with—and eventually marry—a fellow named Tony, another of the proofreaders. He courted her like an expert, the sly dog. I attended their wedding in 1995, bumped into them a couple of times later in various places downtown, and had last seen Tony on his own about 2000 or so. He told me he'd finished law school and was settling into that new career.

"Lainie! Great to see you!" I told her that Thanksgiving Eve. "And how's Tony?"

"He passed away last summer, Joshua."

The worst of it, especially in retrospect, was realizing that she'd expected my question, had been braced for it, so used to hearing it from others for over a year and replying to it resolutely. She was all too prepared for my expression of disbelief, for her necessary recital of the awful facts.

"It was leukemia. They treated him at the Hospital of the University of Pennsylvania. He had a stem-cell transplant and it didn't take, but he gave it all the fight he had, right up to the end. You remember how Tony always was."

Or words to that effect, because the shock her speech provoked made it impossible for those words to sink precisely into my mind, for me to remember them verbatim now. I simply could not believe that Tony was dead, and from a blood cancer similar to my own. I heard it on the sidewalk in front of the neighborhood supermarket and I absolutely would not believe it.

Even worse, Lainie was telling me he'd died in June of the previous year. June 7, 2006, as it turns out, I looked up the obituary online—not two weeks before I entered the same hospital for my own damn transplant. Lainie was Tony's widow now and I couldn't believe it.

Let me tell you about Tony: when he was hired at that awful reporting agency, where I'd already been working for a couple of years, I remembered having seen him before. It had been at a reading sponsored by Temple University's creative writing department in the late 1980s.

There was a noted writer visiting Temple that semester; I was not in the MFA program but only in the audience for one of this author's public readings for which, in order to warm up the crowd, a couple of students had the honor of presenting some of their own work.

To the miked podium came an intense fellow with thick dark hair and five o'clock shadow, a boxer's build, pushing thirty it seemed. There was a resemblance to photographs of the younger Richard Price, or the late actor Cliff Gorman. And this no-nonsense guy read a chunk of manuscript that I still remember—as with Lainie, it is not the exact words I recall but instead the impression. The tone, the aura, a believably tawdry atmosphere in which a man trawled a sex emporium, feeding his quarters into the peepshow slot to make its steel shutter rise upon a naked dancer and, upon the shutter's inevitable prompt fall, more quarters to raise it and raise it again, the man's desperate, bitter conversation with the dancer...

As unpleasant as the story was, it rang honest, the author imparting a section of himself into the pages without apology or undue exhibitionism, unafraid to present that to his readers, the audience impatient to hear from the much more famous writer.

A day came in the office when I worked up the nerve to remind Tony of that evening, and he laughed with no evident embarrassment. He'd stopped writing fiction by then and switched to Temple's film school. He had a tremendous love for the western and war films of the 1950s-70s: Sam Peckinpah, David Lean, Sam Fuller. *Men's* movies, by god! We both loved all those films, and we talked about them all the time.

However, Quentin Tarantino notwithstanding, it transpired that film schools in the 1990s were not hotbeds of support for Charlton Heston enthusiasts, and at some point Tony left the film program, too. But not before I appeared in some test footage he shot one afternoon after work. (Sadly, the world will never witness my searing performance as *Guy Crossing Rittenhouse Square Back and Forth Until Tony Yells "Cut!"*)

We often argued strongly about other passions: music, books, politics, and I like to think we got along as well as we did because each sensed the other's disappointments and compromises. I was happy when he married Lainie, happy he got his law degree and began to make some money.

And here I was, bike helmet topside-down in my palms like a mendicant's perforated bowl, dumbfoundedly listening to Lainie, his *widow,* tell me that that smart burly fellow was dead. This now would be her second Thanksgiving without him.

I kicked myself for not having kept in touch with the pair of them, hating it that the last conversation I'd had with Tony was that bull session in a City Hall concourse where I'd happened to run into him in 2000. He couldn't have been more than two years older than me.

In my disbelief and sadness, I knew one thing: I had to keep my damn mouth shut. *Don't tell her you have myeloma*, I told myself. *Don't tell Lainie how well you're doing with it these days. Keep your goddamn mouth shut.* I had to let Lainie talk. I could not let the conversation tend towards myself. I could not say anything that might upset her any further—and maybe even justifiably anger her, too, force her to wonder, as I wondered then and now, why *I* was still ticking when Tony had succumbed.

No, my job was to stand there and listen. It is all our jobs. Lainie needed badly to talk to someone who'd known her husband. It broke my heart, it breaks it now, to think of how she ran across the street, so eager to see someone she hadn't seen in several years, simply because I'd once known the man she married. And because I'd known him, been fortunate to have intersected in a small way with his life, Lainie could, by talking, get to the bit of Tony left in me. The only decent thing to do was to listen as she said, "Remember the day in the office when Tony did *this*," and "You should have seen the video collection he had in our house, it was a *library*," and, if *I* was to talk at all, it could only be about Tony.

This is the alibi I'm giving myself. This is my excuse for *Marrow Me*, this little me-show I'm putting on: that it's hardly all about me, not at all *my* myeloma. It's lots of people's. Lots of sufferers, too many widows and widowers. Lots of heartbroken people running across the street, desperate to find some trace of their loved ones. They need to be acknowledged, the survivors as much as those who've passed. Because of all the crybaby memoirs out there, there isn't one I know of about myeloma. Because I'm tired of hearing people say "Myeloma? You mean that skin disease?" And because I have to start somewhere, I'm afraid the myeloma story I know best is my own.

Does this make any sense to you? I am writing so I don't have to *talk*.

Chapter Three

ONSET

ALLOWEEN AFTERNOON AT HAWK MOUNTAIN Sanctuary, Kempton, Pennsylvania, the year 2005. Sixty miles northwest of Philadelphia. Black and orange party streamers liven up the Visitors' Center, along with cats, bats and witches crafted from construction paper. Wicked jack-o'-lanterns sit ripe for candling and the onset of night.

This was a Sunday, warm and clear, with a perfectly unclouded sky: first-rate for birding. Hawk Mountain lies directly beneath the Appalachian flyway of migrating North American raptors, and its premier viewing spot is the North Lookout. This is a tremendous heap of exposed rocks, 1500 feet above sea level, left behind by retreating glaciers ten millennia ago (give or take), on which dedicated watchers and official Sanctuary bird counters sit for hours with powerful telephoto equipment. As if by contractual arrangement, vultures, kestrels, falcons, eagles and an extraordinary range of hawks—Red-Tailed and Red-Shouldered, Sharp-Shinned and Rough-Legged—glided over us in succession that day, one after another in review, seeming as high over us as we were over the checker-boarded farms in the valleys below.

There is that particular thrill of catching the speck of bird with your naked eye before fixing it in your viewing device, seeing it spring so close and focused in the lens: the living thing down to its head, eyes and individual feathers, the commanding wingspan that *does not move* even as the bird progresses through the sky. This is the primary thing: the impression of effortlessness, of creatures riding the air without seeming to stir themselves, as if regally bored with the entire commuting process. Literally above it all. The world, spectacularly, beneath their notice. And always solitary: this is what struck me most about them at the time, and what remains most stubbornly in memory now. I saw no mated pairs, no groups, but only each raptor gliding on its own, absent any apparent need for company.

Could they see us, did they watch us watching them? I imagine they studied every one of us sharply, fixing us with their legendary visual powers. What did they make of our mass huddle on the mountain rocks, our glassy-eyed social clump?

In mid-afternoon a great murmur swept through the crowd, fingers pointed, cameras turned: our patience had been rewarded with a bald eagle. There soared the iconic head, the stern yellow beak against its setting of cranial white. The great American herald itself. We watched him glide south all the way out of sight.

I remember these details easily, likely because I have never stopped wondering about that day, wondering how I was able to lie sunny-side up for so long on a broken slab of granite with no aches in my back or ribs. How is that possible? Nothing bothered me that afternoon or even later that night when I returned to Philadelphia and toured the Eastern State Penitentiary, that spectacularly rigged-out "haunted" prison in Fairmount where Miriam worked make-up and the concession stand. Not a hint of twinge. I enjoyed myself, I had fun. Sometimes I think of that Halloween Sunday as the last unstained day. The Treat before the Trick.

Not long after (or perhaps not long before: I didn't take active note of my condition at the beginning, I didn't know it *was* beginning, I wasn't writing everything down), I was jogging along a West Philadelphia sidewalk. It was around the vicinity of 33rd and Chestnut, my hurried pace an effort to catch one of the shuttle buses that run between campuses at the University for which I work, but I had to stop running almost as soon as I began.

Ow, my aching back.

From nowhere came a soreness in my lower spine, a dull hammer stroke with every step, right where the vertebrae join the pelvis. Whoever decided to call this the small of the back? There is nothing small about it, my friends; it contains multitudes.

The shuttle left without me. Not a problem; there is always another one. I was more embarrassed than alarmed about the backache, thinking how out of shape I must be getting, how finally middle-aged. Until then I'd been fairly proud of my physical condition: 44 years old with a tamed waistline and strong set of original teeth, a non-smoker and careful drinker, walking the mile-and-a-half to work every day and back, swimming laps in the University pool three times a week and cycling along the Schuylkill River most weekends, weather permitting. Hair still black, even if in the process of retreating from strategic portions of my scalp like Napoleon abandoning Russia. Vegetarian or nearly. Proud to be not infrequently taken, especially by women, for someone of younger age. So, there is pride, and there is the thing it often goeth before. All I thought was happening to me then, as I stood rubbing my back and watching the shuttle disappear past the 33rd Street Armory, was the onset of midlife pudge, midriff spread, the first obvious signs of physical wear, inevitable and to be accepted.

Not long after that, early November— I know this for certain because I did start writing things down—I began to wake early in the mornings. And earlier and earlier: 4:01, 3:37, 2:59 AM. Dreadful anti-hours described so well in DeLillo's White Noise, marked by the demon-red digits of my clock radio staring me down from the bedside table, brutal prime numbers floating in the dark.

What was I doing awake? I had no particular trouble falling asleep at night. The problem involved staying there.

This became routine. I'd wake at some absurd time and lie on my mattress listening for whatever may have gotten me up, but never heard any sounds, never recalled any terrible dreams. Such a situation is not unique within the human race, of course, and was not new to me, but had never been this bad before. Night after night this consistent waking, and the inability to return to sleep, began to do more than annoy. Chronic fatigue set up camp in my head. There began a downward spiral not unfamiliar from previously snarled patches of my life, fatigue feeding anxiety and crankiness, anxiety feeding the sleeplessness. I struggled to keep from yawning openly during staff meetings, to remain awake at my office desk.

Plus, in the daytime, my back hurt more. There were times when I turned too quickly (or what was never before *too quickly*) and felt an immediate pang in one side or another of my ribcage, sharp and deep. My job often required me to move computers and A/V equipment, to squirm under desks in order to get such gear properly networked, and this was proving more difficult to do without significant trouble. Every once in a while, in my office behind its closed door, I jumped up and down experimentally.

Result of experiment: *ow ow ow*.

The walk to work grew more difficult. I feel I'm dragging myself over the leaf-covered footpaths in Washington Square, get no benefit from the shortcut through Reading Terminal Market, am winded by the time I reach the last blocks I have to cover along the edge of Chinatown. But when I ride the bus or subway, meaning to give myself a break, this only worsens the problem: those goddamn rattletraps, packed with swaying commuters, lurching and jolting over the city's countless potholes and crevasses, play with my spine like the wind plays with chimes. There I am, hanging on to an overhead pole, eyes bugging out with each sudden stop of the transit vehicle.

Something inside of me is wrong.

I remember an interlude from earlier in the year, the first weeks of summer, when I resumed the habit of regular push-ups. I worked up to sets of 50 and more, really getting into it, but finally had to abandon the exercise thanks to a steadily radiating soreness in my right shoulder. A grinding mortar-and-pestle feeling right there in the joint. Another annoying badge of age, I'd figured. But why bother seeing a doctor, when simply quitting the push-ups made the pain go away? And besides (as I considered later in the fall), that was my right shoulder, not my back or ribs. What possible link could there be between my back and ribs and my creaky right shoulder?

Naturally I saw no relation either to the series of head colds that had also commenced in summer, sniffles and scratchy throats and coughing jags settling in and taking longer than usual to leave. Just allergies, right?

Likewise I saw no connection to the epic nosebleed I enjoyed on the sofa one autumn night, while watching the reconstructed version of *The Big Red One* on DVD.

Let me tell you a little about *The Big Red One*: it is a World War Two epic written and directed by Samuel Fuller, originally released in a butchered version of approximately 116 minutes in 1980. In 2004 it was then restored—or "reconstructed," as the promotional material had it—to 158 minutes and re-released in a limited theatrical run for the faithful core of film bugs who'd only ever seen the cropped version on miserable pan-and-scan VHS.

The Big Red One was one of Tom's favorite movies; I hope he managed to see the re-release before he died. When it turned up in the schedule of the Philadelphia Film Festival in May 2005, I got my ticket well in advance; but when the night of the screening actually arrived, I found myself checking the movie's expanded running time against its 9 PM start and weighing that against my post-dinner fatigue and the fact of work the next morning.

Suddenly I wasn't sure I could make it through the movie in one wakeful piece. I biked up to the sold-out theater, paced up and down the line of folks waiting outside, thinking how much I hated to miss the show, but finally decided to sell my ticket to someone in the stand-by line: an elderly gentleman with scarce white hair and a major belly who claimed he really had fought in the Second World War in the Army's First Infantry Division, the actual Big Red One, just like the guys in the movie.

If the man was lying, he did a fine job of it and deserved the ticket anyway. I felt like a responsible citizen and everything, doing a good deed for this combat veteran (or first-class bullshitter) then getting to bed early so as to be at peak working form next day in the office. Besides, the damn thing was coming out soon on DVD anyway, loaded with chewy bonus features, a whole cinematic enchilada I could ingest later at my convenience.

Which, now, I finally was doing, at home, on my sofa, in autumn. Soaking up the exploits of the First Infantry Division (their insignia a large crimson numeral "1," hence the title) as dramatized for the screen by the one-and-only Sam Fuller, who'd served in combat in the division in real life. I watched the cigar-chomping unit fight its colorful way across North Africa and up into Italy, then onto the Normandy beaches and across the rest of Western Europe, led on and growled at and mercilessly goaded by its deathless nameless Sergeant, Lee Fucking Marvin himself.

And as I often do when no one is watching (or, worse, when I *think* no one is watching), I was picking my nose pretty intently. Picking it long past the point where I might have argued to a jury that I was performing any necessary pulmonary maintenance. Let's face it: I was going for broke, prospecting for gold, simply for the tactile pleasure. A ways into the movie I realized my nose was dripping, there in the dark front room of my apartment, in front of the beaming flat screen. And still I didn't react straightaway, didn't bother to pause the movie or even stop my little archeological dig, because this was hardly the first time I had "struck oil," so to speak, while rooting around up there. Such was my swinging bachelor life in the autumn of 2005, sitting home alone with my finger up my nose watching an old war movie in my underwear, an evening so much in the course of routine that I didn't even stop the DVD to examine what was by now dripping onto my undershirt.

It may have been during the movie's unforgettable childbirth scene (a delirious Frenchwoman going into labor inside a tank, her legs up in stirrups rigged from cartridge belts, condoms draped over Lee Marvin's fingers for impromptu gloves, Marvin growling *poussez, poussez*, threatening that baby to come out or else, this whole business taking place right after a major battle, all in all a real showstopper of a sequence) when I realized I was having no ordinary nosebleed but something else entirely. Usually I could get these episodes to end with a couple of quick inward sniffs; usually they dried up on their own. But not this time. There was something warm and constant on my upper lip. A heavy drop patted on my undershirt. Another. I could sense heat, taste salt. All right, I figured: time for a look.

When I got to the bathroom and switched on the light, I saw in the mirror a living slug of blood from my nostril to my lips, even extending well over my upper lip and halfway into my mouth, glossy and only half-coagulated. A big red one! I'd never produced anything like this before. My white undershirt was spotted with the stuff, as if I'd been buckshot. For one shameless moment I allowed myself to think there was something military in my appearance, that I almost resembled one of those soldiers whose story I'd been watching.... except that those guys risked and sometimes lost their lives catching bullets and kicking Nazi ass all the way across Western Europe, while I'd mostly confined myself to picking my nose on the sofa in my underpants.

After admiring myself a while longer, I wiped the mess from my face, threw the spattered shirt in the laundry bag and packed some tissue into the leaky nostril. I don't know why I wasn't more concerned at the time. The bleeding stopped eventually. So what, I must have figured, was the big deal? So, I'd been having some nosebleeds that year...all I needed to do was kick the nose picking habit and there the problem would end, right? What could an escalating series of poorly coagulating nosebleeds possibly have to do with persistent low energy, lingering sinus infections, and chronic back-rib-and-shoulder pain?

But we're well into November now, and nothing's getting better. Certainly not the skeletal problem, particularly in the bullseye of my lower back. And my ribs feel as if they're being "alternatively tuned," like the strings on a Sonic Youth guitar. I like the music, I just don't care to be its instrument. Chronic pings, twinges, pops at any and all times, very alarming.

I was used to severe aches after long hikes and cycle rides, but that's because I was used to them *going away over time*. I was not accustomed to them getting approved for a mortgage and settling in for the duration, bringing in furniture and turning up the surround-sound system. Something was changing inside of me; something was giving way. I could no longer turn at the waist without summoning new types of immediate pain, sharp and eye-widening.

At work, I carefully avoided desk edges and doors, found reasons not to wriggle beneath someone's desk to check their T1 connection or printer cable. Co-workers noticed. They said nothing but I noticed them noticing, frowning at the insomniac smudges beneath my eyes, considering my hunched progress down halls and into my office, where the door was now always closed. At home, even simple acts like lacing my shoes or rinsing a pot required careful planning.

I recall one fizzled date I had about this time, during the entirety of which I couldn't stop rubbing my right arm. What woman could fail to be turned on?

Anyone suffering ill-health learns that one thing you're likely to do is to pull back further into yourself, and I am no exception. I paid increasingly less attention to the world and its calamities: drowned New Orleans in the continued afterwash of Katrina; the broadening fiasco of the American occupation of Iraq, the country burning and bleeding every 100-degree-plus day, US troop deaths edging over 2,000; Vice-Presidential aide Scooter Libby charged with obstruction of justice in the Valerie Plame case; killer tornadoes in the Midwest (22 dead), weeks of civil riots in France, bombings in Delhi (61 dead), bombings in Amman (at least 50 dead), details I have to search for today in news archives in order to know them, in order to get them straight. In autumn 2005, disease has softened my bones but heightened my selfishness: How can I care about anyone else's death and destruction when my back hurts *so much?*

Because that, of course, is what's been hauling me out of Dreamsville every night. My back doesn't retire when I go to sleep. My back is wide awake all the time now, it's up all night and wants to be kept company. No more of this nudging me awake subliminally. Now my back says: *You and I need to talk.* It says: *I'm up so* you're *going to be up too, and you're going to stay up.* There's no hope of moving into a more comfortable position in bed, because there is no such thing as a comfortable position anymore. I don't even dare to take a deep breath. Hours of ginger mattress-misery pass, and at last the bedroom window begins to lighten, the signal for me to officially rise, to "wake," every morning now the same extended process: several minutes of timid wriggling while I force one limb and then another closer to the edge of the bed, angling my legs out and over for support, both hands on the night table for support, an unwelcome version of Twister to start every goddamn day. I can't suppress groans, helpless little screams as I force myself upright. I am certain my closest neighbors in my apartment building formed an entirely inaccurate impression of my morning activities during this period.

Something had to be done.

There was a "relaxation sanctuary" in my neighborhood, a low-key spa offering therapeutic massage, meditative baths and the like. I'd passed it countless times without a thought of entering. But I'd been reminded of it recently: every Halloween, the managers staged clever skits behind their bay window and on the sidewalk in front of it, delighting local children and adults both. This most recent Halloween, the night of the day of the hawks, they'd done a goof on *Jurassic Park*, the staff miming hilariously in cheap safari costumes, one guy in a handmade T-rex outfit assaulting the others, rubber limbs tossed around for gory laughs, a plastic pterodactyl dangling from a second-floor window. Just the place to go for some serious medical attention.

Under better circumstances, I would have enjoyed the Saturday hour I spent there. There was calm and stillness in the massage room on the second floor, scented candles and drawn shades and a CD's-worth of narcotized ambience, all the things I've slowly learned over time not to sneer at so immediately. The therapist, an athletic blonde woman about my age, was professionally skilled, and, yes, not unappealing in her general ministrations. But, through no fault of hers, I left more frightened than when I arrived. Lying down on the padded table was a trial, with much flinching and grunting and gnashing of the teeth. When the therapist applied herself to certain portions of my back, I yelled and begged her to quit. When she asked me to roll from one side to another, I cried out again as I moved, however slowly. I felt ashamed in front of this woman and scared of the worried looks she gave me.

To her great credit, she said, "There's something wrong with you that I can't fix."

She didn't give me any mumbo-jumbo about chakras or energy fields or try to tell me I needed exclusive care that only her spa could provide. Instead she recommended over-the-counter pain medication (*bonjour*, little white bottle of Motrin!), muscle liniment, and perhaps I ought to think about seeing a chiropractor.

Of course! A chiropractor! Why didn't I think of that before? Now we'll get to the bottom of this spinal business! I had become fixated on the thought (the *hope*) that all my troubles might be traced to one concentrated spot in my lower back, some nexus of bone, muscle and nerve, bollixed-up in a Gordian knot which some skillful manipulator could undo with a single skilled rap of the knuckles, as simple as slipping a key into a lock. I had even come to imagine the sweet sound this release might make, a moist crack of the vertebrae followed by instantaneous relief. People I spoke to around this time told me stories not far removed from this fantasy. Co-workers, cabdrivers, supermarket clerks: *My back/shoulder/ribs were in horrible shape, I couldn't stand up in the morning, but then this guy I saw pressed right on this one point and I'm telling you, I practically danced out of his office!*

It didn't happen that way. I made an appointment with a chiropractor, one within limping distance of my home. A foolish reason to choose a doctor, certainly, just because she's conveniently located, but I felt I might as well give my bones as easy a time as possible—not to mention this clinic was covered by my insurer.

She was intrigued and carefully attentive but could not prevail against whatever it was my back was turning into or had already become. At my first visit, she took a brief history, said it all sounded familiar to her and she was sure she could bring me some relief, but as with the relaxation spa, the simple act of lying face-down on her examination table was a production in itself. I can still see the look on the chiropractor's face: *Well, this is a challenge.* I sensed her annoyance, not with me so much as with a situation that refused to come right.

What I remember best from these sessions is the acquaintance I made of the doctor's Transcutaneous Electrical Nerve Stimulation (TENS) unit, a device she hauled out towards the end of my first appointment. The unit looked dubious, early lo-tech, like some piece of A/V equipment that might have been used in my elementary school, back when dinosaurs roamed the earth: a black plastic box with painted dials, and two wriggly electric cords ending in white pads. I sit in an open-backed chair while the doctor sticks the pads on my bared lower back, after slathering me there with gel. Then she turns a dial on the box.

"How does that feel?"

"Could you put the pads a little lower?"

"Here?"

"Oh yeah, that's it." There's a steady humming against my skin, a strong current of resistance. For the first time in weeks I experience a hint of genuine relief. Finally, someone understands, even if it is only an electric pad.

"All right," the doctor says, "I'm turning it up. How's that?"

"More."

"Okay, I'm turning it up."

"More."

"You want more?"

"More." I'm beginning to feel something like relief. "Does it go any higher?"

The chiropractor has come around to look me in the eye. She does not seem overly pleased.

"That's as high as it goes."

"Really? Is there another one you could put on?"

"No. And it's pretty rare for the setting to be this high."

"Can I take this one home? Where do you buy one of these things?"

Chapter Four

SCANNERS

T HE CHIROPRACTOR IS NICE, BUT the relief I'm getting is only temporary. For an hour or so after I leave, I feel like there's some progress, but it's only skin deep and by bedtime I'm easing myself into bed as gingerly as ever, and the mornings seem worse. I don't wake up, I am jolted up.

I make an appointment with my primary care physician.

I'm taking Motrin, rubbing liniment on my back, keeping my spine straight at all times, trying to perform the at-home exercises prescribed by the chiropractor. None of it is any help. I'm still having trouble carrying simple things. My shoulder pack I use for work weighs more each day. I can't bend to lift anything anymore: I have to squat, use the knees, as if I'm herniated. I've got new aches now, my stomach muscles because of the way I'm holding myself, trying to keep my back out of it.

Thanksgiving dinner at my older sister's house in Bucks County. I'm loaded with ibuprofen. It's fun, and the food is great, and I'm able to hide my condition. Mom, and Dad with Parkinson's since spring 2001, his right hand at an angle, fingers pressed together, endlessly shaking, as if motioning to an invisible waiter, endlessly signaling "bring the check, bring the check, bring the check..."

My younger sister, Judith, is there with her son and daughter, and the boy is two years old and running around and he wants to be lifted and I can't lift him. Somehow my parents don't notice my back, got to keep them from noticing. But when I'm sitting on the sofa and my nephew runs up and wants to play I have to wave him off, and his father, my brother-in-law—who just happens to work in orthopedic research—notices. I make excuses. Bad back, and so on.

But my older sister, the nurse practitioner at FCCC, gives me a ride to the Neshaminy Falls rail station. We're early and it's cold out so I sit in the van and talk as we're waiting for the train to come in, and I start telling her about my back. Telling her I've got a doctor's appointment for the next Monday. Cancer hasn't even crossed my mind. It's back pain, remember. What can back pain possibly have to do with cancer, how or why would you even think of cancer?

I am still riding my bicycle during this period, but riding is not the problem, it's the mounting and dismounting that are killing me. I can feel things shifting, popping, sliding as I maneuver on and off the bike.

The Friday after Thanksgiving. The big break. I recall I went to a movie that afternoon, either *Capote* or *The Squid and the Whale*, one of those movies that came out around that time and made the writing life look especially toxic. Most of the day is lost to me. November 25: puttering around apartment. Trying to get into bed. All I want to do is get into bed, lie on my back and get to sleep. But any little bit of pressure on the back seems insupportable. Moving to the left, to the right, leaning backwards. I just can't ease into it. I'm looking for that zone, that spot....

I turn on my right side to get up out of bed, and as my feet touch the floor I experience what, just under three weeks later, an MRI scan will confirm is a vertebral fracture (the first of two I will enjoy). That is, I break a bone in my lower spine simply by moving to stand.

Allow me to elaborate upon that sensation. Try to recall the best orgasm you ever had, or at least one of the best. Perhaps it was fortunately recent, a real body-melting wave germinating in your core and radiating to your extremities. Wasn't it good? Try and imagine it lasting for six or seven minutes. Even better, right? Now, bearing that all in mind, try and reverse the impression so that, rather than the flooding of all your pleasure receptors, your nerves are instead overwhelmed by the same intensity of pain. A six or seven-minute paingasm. Yeah, that's about what I remember it feeling like. I often wish I had a tape recording of those six or seven minutes, in order to have the pleasure of destroying it. I know that any neighbors who may have overheard had to believe I was having the time of my sexual life.

I remember falling forward into my bureau holding myself up on my forearms, wondering what was happening. I remember struggling to keep my weight off my legs because I was afraid they would not support me, thinking I had broken my spine and/or was otherwise paralyzed, afraid that if I fell to the floor I would not be able to rise. Six or seven minutes.

Eventually the first wave of sensation rolled back. I had to try to walk sometime. I lifted one foot, set it down, lifted the other. Locomotion. Wiggled toes. What do you know: not paralyzed. It looked likely that I would even be able to make my way over to the bedside table an entire 18 inches to my right, and to the jar of painkillers (ibuprofen) there, if I was extra-cautious. That's what I did. Very, very slowly, without lifting a foot this time but rather sliding over the wooden floor, I maneuvered to the table, arms on the bureau all the while, until I was close enough to reach down and grab the bottle. How laughable and pathetic it seems now, that non-prescription bottle.... Oh, little non-prescription bottle, where are you now? How fearlessly you tried to help. I worked three capsules out and swallowed them dry, stood there another quarter of an hour until they began to take effect. Then I began to move again, not walking but moving, slithering over the floor into the front room of my apartment. I knew something was terribly wrong. I was fighting panic and it was a close thing. I didn't know how I was ever going to lie on my back again, that evening or ever. I did not know if the pain would subside, if I should call an ambulance, if I would spend that night or subsequent nights in the hospital, if EMTs would momentarily be stomping up the stairs and into my rooms. There was in all this one thought predominant in my mind:

I have to clean up my mess.

As I stated, I really thought I was broken that night. Really thought I would be out of commission for a good while, laid up, packed away somewhere out of my apartment while other people came in and out to get necessary things. Other people would likely need access to my laptop for files, or failing that would have to get my laptop and bring it to me and could I trust them not to turn the machine on in the meantime, boot it up and maybe look at files in my absence? Nope, no question about it.

I sit in my swivel chair and watch my legs twitch uncontrollably for minutes. Apparently, this is muscle tension relaxing. What is wrong with me? I was an idiot not to have gone to an emergency room. What did I think I was doing, holding out till Monday's doctor appointment?

The next day, Thanksgiving Saturday, I actually attend a Philadelphia Orchestra concert. Beethoven's Third. Somehow I take public transit into the center of town, riding the bus, the subway. I remember sweating a lot, but somehow being able to deal with the situation. The events of the previous night seemed only a sort of lapse, a momentary break in routine. Never did it occur to me that I'd broken anything inside, that I might be walking around with some sort of permanent fracture. Besides, I was seeing the doctor on Monday. Why rush things? He'd take a look at me and tell me what was wrong.

In other words, I was a complete idiot.

So, Monday comes around. Heading into the doctor's office for an appointment beats going to work any day, right? Only guess what? I'm more nervous than I think, and what do I do when I'm nervous?

That's right, pick my nose.

I'm sure none of the other waiting patients notice a thing, especially when I strike oil in my left nostril and the red drip starts and just won't stop. Nosebleed City. I sniff and inhale and sniff. I wipe frantically with a paper tissue. I shove a wad of tissue up there, like some boxer, like Philadelphia's own Rocky Balboa, and hope nobody notices the crimson rat's-tail of sopping tissue hanging from the center of my face.

I get up and check myself in the restroom mirror. Delicately tug out the tissue. Okay, the bleeding has finally stopped. What I'm left with, I discover as I tilt my head back, is a small but living moist red blob parked in my nostril, like a grandchild of the one Steve McQueen battled in the film of the same name (the original setting of *The Blob* was nearby me, out in the suburbs of Philadelphia, as it happens—Phoenixville, PA, back in 1958). If I breathe too heavily through my nose, the thing quivers dangerously, ready to flow again, so it's mouth-breathing time in the lobby.

Here comes a nurse. I am weighed and measured, then directed to an examination room, and when my doctor comes in, my GP, Doctor S

(1) (because there are two more Doctor Ss), I start laying it on the line. The back pain, the back pain, the back pain. I don't say a word about the other things, the things I do not realize are symptoms, because I do not realize they are symptoms. The colds. The fatigue. The nosebleeds. I mean, the fatigue, of course I'm fatigued, with this back pain who wouldn't be fatigued, who can sleep with this shit.

Dr. S1 takes my history, and I remember he does something specific. First, he asks me to lie down on the examination table. I refuse.

"I'm afraid to lie down. I can't lie down."

Okay, no worries, don't lie down.

I have my shoes still on, and he cups one foot in his hands and tells me to push down as hard as I can. I do that, and he repeats with the other foot.

Okay. Good. Strong. In his Russian accent.

I know he's checking for damage to my spinal cord, whether there might be impingement on nerves there, whether I still have control of the lower portion of my body.

"Any pains in your legs?"

"No."

"Any weakness?"

"No."

"Very good. Let's look at the rest of you."

The good doctor looks in my eyes, he looks in my ears. You know what's coming. He's got his little lighty-scope and he's looking up my nostrils.

"Mr. Roberts, I am seeing some obstruction in your nostril."

Ah ha ha ha. Really, you don't say. And I'm so mortified that I actually explain the quivering blood-booger up there, explaining how while I was sitting in the waiting room, or waiting in the sitting room, I was, ah ha ha, just trying to, ah, clear, yeah, that's it, clear my nose a little, just anybody else would, and ah, heh heh, went a little too far, it seems. Sorry about that.

The doctor smiles understandingly and advises that the next time I feel like clearing my nose, I might want to think about simply blowing into a Kleenex. I'm about as humiliated as I've ever been in my life... though this standard will prove short-lived and will be broken again and again over ensuing months, you wait and see.

We make the quantum jump up the painkiller rungs: a prescription for Darvocet.

So, I'm sent down the hall for standard blood work and a flu shot, which fortunately is the killed virus since the live one might have killed me, given my lack of immune function. Then it's across the street, to Jefferson Hospital's radiology department, for a back x-ray. To my surprise, no appointment is needed for one of these; you just show up and wait your turn. This seems wonderfully egalitarian at first until after two hours go by and I'm sick of waiting. But they finally get me in there, stripped to the waist and in my gown, and I lean against the big boxy panel on the wall and let the camera snap away.

Then I head into the office and pretend to work for the rest of the day.

Of course, I'm still going to my own chiropractor, which is where I am (Wednesday night, November 30) when the call comes on my cell. I'm hooked up to the TENS unit and life is momentarily fine. It's a clinician from the radiology department (or was it someone from my GP's office?), a young Asian woman by the sound of her voice, and she has the results of my x-ray, and they are not good. Advanced osteoporosis. I'm sitting there in the chiropractor's office, cell phone to my head, TENS unit electro sticky pads on my back, trying to make sense of the call.

"Osteoporosis?" Like what little old ladies have?

"Yes, Mr. Roberts, and the x-ray shows it is not confined to the area of your lower back. It is pervasive throughout all featured bones, and it is advanced."

"Oh great."

The chiropractor, I clearly recall, laughs at my reaction. Is this her way of trying to ease the tension, deflate the situation, by turning it all into a joke?

I spend the waking part of the next 24 hours or so pondering this question. How can I have osteoporosis? This simply makes no sense. How can I have little old lady bones? It's the lactose intolerance, I decide, that's what it is. All those years of avoiding milk. Calcium deficiency. I pledge to buy calcium tablets by the crate, to wear bandoliers of Lactaid tablets over my shoulders at all times in order that I may eat dairy products at every meal. I'll move to a farm and suck milk straight from a cow's teats. Whatever it takes to get rid of this miserable flaming back that now flares up and hurts more than ever.

But next afternoon I have something else to worry about. Dr. S1 calls me at work and he has something to tell me.

"Joshua, I am looking at your blood tests and of course I also have the results of your x-rays. I am a little concerned and I am thinking you need to have some more blood tests and we need to x-ray more of your body. We need to rule things out, but I have a concern that you may have myeloma."

"Oh yeah? What's that?"

If there's any conversation out of this entire experience that I have trouble recollecting in detail, it's this one. I won't even try to recreate dialogue here: it's paraphrase time again. I was completely disoriented and scatter minded, exactly as I believe anyone is who begins to hear news like this about himself or a loved one. Myeloma? I have a disease now? It has a name? What I've got is so bad that it has a name? A disease? Come on, I know I have a bad back but a bad back isn't a disease. How can I have a disease? I don't have a disease. It's my back that's giving me problems, not a disease. Fix my back, will ya? What kind of disease gives you a bad back?

Well, I'm beginning to find out. Naturally once my conversation with the good doctor is over, I begin to research information on myeloma on the faultless repository of all things known to man, aka the Internet.

Actually, because I work for a health school within a large University, I have access to all sorts of medical databases, actual medical literature, mostly inaccessible to the general public. This is one of the few good breaks I get: I'm piped in to the good stuff. I look up general definitions before I get until the serious medical databases to which my job allows me access.

So here's where I find out that it's a form of cancer. I don't remember what sources I used for this all-important information. Did I look at peer-reviewed articles first, or did I go straight to Google and Wikipedia like any other chump?

What kind of cancer causes a bad back? That's right: myeloma. Turns out back pain (and related pain in other weight-bearing bones) is one of the primary symptoms presented by patients who end up being diagnosed with the disease.

And what is multiple myeloma a cancer of? The blood system, specifically a type of white blood cell called the "plasma cell."

I simply don't recall if Dr. S1 used the word *cancer* in our phone conversation or not. I just have the general recollection that he tried as calmly and soothingly as possible to give me the required information without raising any undue alarm. I still don't know what other diseases my initial tests might have pointed to, what else I might have possibly had, what possibilities needed to be eliminated. But all I remember hearing is the word myeloma, the possibility of myeloma, and nothing about cancer.

This, by the way, is why it often helps to have someone trustworthy along when you have a doctor for a serious medical consultation. They'll often remember the things that can't, the things you're too stunned to absorb.

I know I have a bad back and it needs some tending to, but a disease? So, I can only give you the gist: that I make an appointment to meet the doctor again, with the knowledge that I'm heading into some serious tests: a second more detailed round of blood work, urine testing, full body x-rays and an MRI. An MRI? That's for sick people!

I genuinely don't remember Dr. S1 at that time explaining in any detail what myeloma is, the likelihood of my having it, or anything like that. He was actually being quite a good doctor, putting it in terms of elimination, that I might have myeloma but quite possibly not, that I'm just passing along to another stage of examination. Nothing etched in stone yet, nothing determined, we just need to look a little closer.

It's a good thing I've been taking that Darvocet, because on top of making my back endurable it also keeps me sedated to a degree. So I'm only panicking a little.

Cancer. Blood cancer. But of course, this can't be true. I have a bone problem, not cancer. I have a backache problem, not cancer. Even as I read some of the symptoms—elevated protein levels, bone ache, back pain—I'm still in denial. I see some other stats: a disease of the elderly (hits people in their 60s), statistically higher in black Americans than whites. So, it's got to be something else, right?

It all gets to be sort of a blur. I phone my older sister and tell her what the doctor said. This is the critical point. I don't remember what is said, but the critical thing is that Margot insists she be placed on speed dial, in effect—put in the loop, kept up to date. I insist that our parents not be told, not till everything is cleared up.

Cleared up, ha. Made definite, I guess, is what I meant.

Dr S1 comes through and gets me an appointment for early next week, the week of December 5th. He fixes me up with a bunch of referrals and prescriptions: a big bunch of blood tests, a urine test, then I have to get an MRI. I get directed to the lab my primary care office uses—another one of those places where there's no appointment, you just kind of wander in and take a number. When it's my turn they take vial after vial. Hey, leave me something to get home with, will you? I tell them I'm on serious prescription painkillers and ask if this will have any effect on the tests. No. No? I'm pumped full of painkillers and won't have any effect on medical tests? What if I was drunk? Can't you test me for drugs instead of cancer?

They give me an enormous brown plastic jug. What's this?

"That's for your urine sample."

I look at the thing. It's like a half-gallon.

"You expect me to fill this thing up? Haven't you got anything smaller?"

"No, this is for your 24-hour urine collection. You're going to take this container home with you. We need you to collect all the urine you produce within a 24-hour period. The rule is you start in the morning, only you don't collect your first urination of the day. You flush that. Thereafter you will collect, into this container, all the urine you produce that day. The following morning, 24 hours later, you collect that first urine production. Oh, and one other thing."

"Yeah?"

"You need to keep the container refrigerated."

"What? You expect me to keep this piss jug in the fridge? For how long?"

"All during the collection process, Mister Roberts."

"You expect me to keep a jug full of piss in my fridge for 24 hours? Are you out of your mind? I'm trying to get better, not make myself sicker."

I am given a clear plastic sack, the sort used for disposal of medical waste. There's even a biohazard symbol printed in blue on the plastic.

"Keep the jug inside of this while you're collecting."

"Sure, that'll do the trick. All the food in my fridge will know to keep a safe distance from the jug, what with the clearly stated warning on the bag and all. I just hope that the milk and the mustard and the bread have time to read the warning in full before the fridge door shuts and the light goes out. You never really know what goes on in there after the door closes and the light goes out."

My comedy routine is not making much of an impression on the staff.

"Okay, for real now, how soon do you need this?" Because it's dawning on me as well that I don't know how I can do this collection in the course of a work day. I can't bring a jug of piss into work, carry it in and out of the office restroom when I need to relieve myself, and store it in the office fridge in the downtime. Even I know that this is socially unacceptable.

It's the middle of the week. I can't be dealing with the mechanics of a jugful of urine in and out of the fridge at work. And it doesn't even occur to me (though it will in future) that I can take a sick day off work simply to urinate at home.

"Can you wait until Monday? Can you wait for me to collect this Sunday and I'll bring it in Monday?"

"As soon as possible." But I detect no great personal urgency on their part, and I begin to notice what all patients notice: they've got other patients to concentrate on in the lab. The inevitable result of dealing with great numbers of people is that I am not the main focus of their day. That in the end it devolves to me, my decisions, that I am on my own. I can choose to bring in the urine whenever I want, I can choose not to bring it in at all, I can choose never to see another doctor again...and I won't be particularly missed, because there's no shortage of patients to take up the lab technicians' time, the doctors' time. This is reality.

December 7: the day of the long-bone survey. Good title for a book! Somehow, I shuffle over to the hospital for the big event. Why didn't I take a cab? Punishing myself. Wanting to see how much of this business

I could take. Only invalids take cabs to go a few blocks. I don't take a cab to go a few blocks, ergo I am not an invalid.

This time it's serious. This isn't a passport photo, this is the full wedding album. I have to strip to my underwear, put on a full hospital gown like an inpatient. I lie on a glass tabletop. I've got to maneuver from one side to another and I need assistance. Guess I am an invalid. The lab techs have to help me on and off the table. They are very considerate and patient about it; I expect they have some experience.

Don't tell the parents, don't tell the parents, don't tell the parents.

It's murder having to shift from one side to the other. Visions of my elders as I move my groany bones in my gown, my scrawny body exposed and feeble and helpless.

***

THERE IS A MULTICULTURAL DINNER at my house on the night of December 8. I borrow some computer equipment from the university so I can put on a digital slide show. What was I thinking, hauling that shit around? A student has to help me haul the case up and down the stairs.

There's snow that night, and then I have to deal with getting the equipment back to work the next morning. Slush-covered sidewalks, the wheels on the case won't roll, the wheel mechanisms jamming with slush. I'm not wheeling the thing, I'm dragging it.

I'd stay home, but there's a panel at work on the aftermath of Hurricane Katrina. I'm the guy who helps set these things up, gets the cables and PowerPoints in place, and makes sure everyone's online and wired and miked and ready to go, so I have to be there. Try to get a cab in my neighborhood on a slushy morning—not going to happen. I finally get a taxi, and the driver has to throw the case in the trunk. I tell him about my bad back and even he's got advice for me. Everyone's got advice.

Setting up for American Public Health Association that week. My back problems are obvious; I can't hide them from co-workers. Simply carrying a laptop in a shoulder bag is too much. Always so tired.

So the weekend comes, with Sunday on tap (so to speak) for urine collection. What do female cancer patients do? Doesn't seem fair for them. What sort of a day was that Sunday...I don't recall the day so much, how often I left the apartment, how far I went when I did. But after a couple of times I begin to enjoy the collection. I'm such a bad boy. Almost taking pride: wow, look how much urine. Is it a sign of health that I'm pissing this much? Or is it bad? Screwing that lid on tight, sliding it into the giant encompassing plastic bag, placing it back on the bottom shelf of the fridge, so if it leaks it won't hit anything.

I'm not super big on noting things down; at least not at that time I wasn't. How much urine I produced, and so forth. Surely this was just one peculiar stage, an unusual event why bother taking notes, what kind of weirdo takes notes about pissing into a jug? I'm not going to be doing this on a routine basis, right?

The next morning, Monday, is cold, chill, cold enough for me to take the jug back to the lab without a cooler. I put the whole thing, jug and plastic wrapper, in a brown grocery sack, and tote it with me out into the refrigerated world. I'm afraid to get on public transit with the thing, afraid of being found out, of having it spill in public, so I walk. Better it spills on the sidewalk, near a gutter, than in a subway car or taxi. But that turns out to be the hard part, because the jug has acquired some weight. What am I doing, shuffling across downtown with my aching back and a heavy bag that, more than once a city block, I shift from one hand to the other....

I'm happy to drop it off at the lab: a kid at his first day at school. I feel like I accomplished something, like I'm making some sort of progress, like I've put something behind me. Turned a corner. One less thing to worry about. All I've got left to worry about now is the MRI on Thursday. Then we'll get to the bottom of things, right?

Naturally, that week, everything collapses quickly and entirely. Tuesday morning, I wake to back pain so miserable I have to take a day off, call in sick. The back has utterly collapsed. I don't believe I can leave the apartment, make it down the stairs, let alone into the office. I can't bend; the only time I feel relatively comfortable is when I sit. I can feel things moving in there. I cannot sleep. I am dead tired and I cannot sleep. The Darvocet isn't doing much. A deep cough has settled into my chest, the likes of which I have not seen since the great bronchitis bout of the summer of '99. It's not enough that I'm bringing up big gummy bears of tapioca-worthy mucus. It's that hair-trigger back, too. Every time I cough I really cough, and my back is forced to bend and shake; the fact is I am breaking apart. Each round of coughing feels like the heel of a karate hand thumping my lower back. In the afternoon

I'm loading clothes in the washer when the fit comes on, and I have to hold on to the machine for support, still coughing so hard that the open jug of detergent falls from the shaky machine and spills over the basement floor. Very cinematic.

There's one other problem, too. When I call Dr. S1's office, to see if the test results are in yet, I'm told that he's away for several days. Nice of him to let me know. I know he's got a life and everything but come on, you big cancer-tease, don't leave me dangling like this.

Earlier I compared my bones to oddly re-strung wires. New metaphor coming up! A decayed sailing ship. That's right. I no longer have a skeletal system. My skeleton, my bones, have long since departed. In its place is a wooden sailing ship, and the masts and the spars are worm-eaten and raw, and the sails are torn away, and the sea is high and the wind higher, and a storm is raging and I am draped over it, I am the sails. A gale is in effect, gale force warning, and I am lost at sea, and I fear the masts are beginning to snap, they creak and are threatening to snap. Someone is screaming, the wind or me, into the teeth of the gale. No sight of land, land is long gone, the sky is black and impenetrable, blind reckoning, there is no way to know where to steer.

On Wednesday, I figure I can't stay at home forever. I'm beginning to worry about the future, and how this is looking to my employers. Out of work for how many days on account of a bad back? Boy, am I going to get in trouble. I fortify myself with Darvocet and head off to work.

Forget about walking. It's public transit for me, hanging on the poles and supports for dear life as the bus finds every goddamn pothole to bounce over, lousy fucking goddamn Philadelphia streets, as the subway lurches in and out of stops. I make it through all that just so that I can get into the lobby of my building and fail.

Another deep horrible tickle hits the back of my throat and I cough hugely and it feels like a mule kicks my spine out from under me. The only reason I don't fall flat out on the floor is that the woman beside me, waiting as I am for the elevator, catches hold of me as I sink and bears me up. She helps me waddle over to the security desk where the guard eyes me like a bouncer and I'm a drunk.

"Back gone out?" he asks casually.

I can barely speak, cannot stand straight, am terrified to be falling apart in public, in front of people I know, people I see every day. I claw another cough drop out of my bag and clamp it in my mouth. A cough has undone me. The cough that won't go away.

I call my boss on my cell phone and explain how once again I won't be coming into work, even though I made it as far as the lobby. Somehow word has filtered up into the office as to my dramatic lobby performance, and Miriam comes down, bearing her chiropractic contact. I don't know what to do. Could it just be that I just need one experienced twist from a chiropractor? One little karate chop and whatever is displaced down there will pop back into its ordered place and I'll let out one gigantic sigh of satisfaction, like that cab driver said? I know I can't get to my chiropractor right now, and so maybe this is the guy to see.

I fall into a cab and get myself driven to 16th and Walnut, take the elevator to the chiropractic office.

The visit is a disaster.

The chiropractor, I can see, is a considerate fellow, genuinely concerned and wanting to help. But from the instant I try to lie upon his table—a process that takes several minutes—I am in further agony. I'm on my side, and the man presses his palms against my hips. Merely lays his hands on my hips, and I cry out. My mind is a rat in a hot wheel. Panic panic panic. I am falling apart and I know it. I am in a bad way and it is only getting worse.

The good man tries to apply some pressure, says he's going to try popping my disc back into alignment or something like that. But as soon as he makes the first attempt, puts his hands on me, I am crying out, begging him to stop. Then it comes, the big emotional breakdown, the total fucking pussy that I have become breaks down and wails right there in the treatment room, bursts into tears and weeps like a baby. Breaks down like his skeleton and wails, and as I recall it, even wails biblically, as in "What is happening to me?" or something like that. I have finally slipped over some sort of edge and I know it.

I have to get off that table. I can't move. I can't move because every time I move it feels like I'm about to break inside. It's not an ache now, we're well beyond ache, we're into pain. I'm scared, I recall the panic

I've seen in the eyes of animals—horses, cats, dogs, whether strays or pets—the panic of being cornered or sick or in incomprehensible pain.

I recall a walk in the woods with my father and a stray cat howling and stalking us from out behind some trees. Why it came to us when you'd expect it to run away I can't imagine, and I don't know how old I was but even then I could see that the red open angry stump where its tail should have been was the result of deliberate mutilation.

I hear it now, and I have heard screaming like that on hospital floors and from behind clinic doors, and that day and moment it came from me. The helpless panic, the tears. The incomprehensibility. And to top it off came the tickle in the back of my throat, the inescapable maddening tickle that means a cough. I know what the cough means, and I can't prevent it, it's a real ragged Devil's Island cough coming on, and it hits, and I go into convulsions, my back arcs again and the pain is more than I can bear.

The chiropractor backs off. He's looking at me like I've grown a third arm, a second head. Like he's never seen anything like me before. So, it really is bad, it really is bad, I think as I slither off the table, snakewise, octopus-out-of-the-ocean wise, helpless, deboned, more frightened than I've ever been in my life.

The look of the chiropractor. What he says, mirroring what the masseuse said: There's something wrong with you. I can't help you. I pull myself up, there's the interlude where I feel the cough coming on and the doctor holds me steady, keeping my back steady till the spasm passes. I am completely helpless. The man has essentially told me there is nothing he can do.

All I can do is pop another Darvocet and stand (because I'm afraid to sit) in the waiting room until it kicks in enough for me to tiptoe out and call a cab. I am now officially scared to death. I am afraid to sit, I am afraid to lie down, I am afraid to stand. It hangs in my mind that I am scheduled for an MRI early the next morning, and even through my painkiller haze I fear the simple act of lying down. The requirement of lying down scares me, the terrifying fact that lying down will be necessary.

I get out of the cab in a junkie blur, everything hideously wrong. It is bright noon, it is midday, I should not be at this place at this hour, creeping out of the back of a cab in front of my apartment building, drug-dazed at noon, a rockstar without any of the fun. *Everything is wrong.* I don't remember much, beyond the exhaustion that keeps me from remembering much. The fatigue didn't allow anything to sink in.

At some point I get into bed. I haven't figured out yet how to sleep upright in a chair or on the sofa (that will come later) and I remember nearly crying for sleep. Dopey, exhausted, scared of myself, scared of what was going on then and more scared of what was to come. I remember being more scared of the prospect of lying down and staying down in the MRI device for an hour, than of having to see my doctor.

But at some point, I looked at my bed and like someone looking at delicious food to which he has a terrible allergy, I couldn't resist. I just needed to lie down. And by bits and degrees—*I might as well get used to it,* I think, *I'm going to have to do this tomorrow*—by leaning this way and that, by keeping my back straight while sort of easing myself down on my right side, I make it into bed, where I promptly fall asleep for several hours.

When I wake, I'm paralyzed. The bedside lamp is still on, and outside the evening has come, and everything is different and I can't move. I'm on my right side in the classic fetal position, and my arms and legs won't move, I can feel them but they are locked in position and don't want to move.

Help. Everything that was worse has just gotten worse.

I try bouncing myself a little bit, and whatever it was, momentary paralysis or whatever, it ends. My joints work. Maybe it was some sort of dream residue, because nothing like this has ever happened since.

But I suppose that I overcompensate, and in my haste to get out of this, to get out of bed, I move too quickly to sit up. For the second time, what feels like a molten wire plunges into my back and twists. A repeat performance of what I don't know yet is a cracked vertebra.

I believe I break my previous screaming record. Oddly I am in the same position as last time, propped up on the bedroom bureau, all my weight on my arms. Attempting to press the thing through the floor, too wildly scared to put my weight on my legs for fear they will not work or bear me up. My body must like something about this position.

Everything just gets worse. Yes, I suppose this was the worst day of my life. The whole process repeats: the slow relaxation down to tippy toes, the allowance of deeper breaths, the very very slow walk on tiptoe to the side table and the painkillers, the test walk out to the front room, the collapse into my swivel chair. I am now well over the maximum dose of painkillers.

At some point I call my older sister to report on events. I remember telling her I didn't think I could go through with the MRI, her saying that was ridiculous, that of course I had to. I remember calling my friend Tim who lives close by, but not whether I spoke to him in person or left a message, but something to the effect that I feared I was being crippled, that I might need his help very soon and very often. I know I took a pillow from the sofa and fell asleep at my desk, sitting at my swivel chair, keeping my back as erect as possible, my head resting on the two pillows.

I will not sleep in a bed for five months.

Which is where pre-dawn finds me, December 15, awake and still dopey. There must have been something like sleep in there, at some point, because eventually I lifted my head from the pillow and found the room faintly lighter. Those hours again, the low-cost figures of pre-dawn: 2:49. 3:50. 5:25. How could I have imagined I might miss the MRI appointment? I could wake up the doctors.

It's dim in my mind now, dim as the light was. I don't know how many Darvocets I took but it was more than recommended. I didn't have to bother getting dressed because I'd never undressed. I knew I'd never undress again. This was the state of my disease. The unwashed jeans, the flannel shirt, the decaying boots I walked in in Vietnam and Cambodia. I will dress no more forever.

MRI: outside slowly into the slowly raising light. Momma always taught me to be early for an MRI. Finding a cab easily has always been an advantage in my neighborhood, and it was as easy that morning. The trick was getting into the cab. The next trick was getting out of it again. I have to tell the driver to please not drive so fast, to please avoid the most broken sections of these godamned downtown Philadelphia streets, on account of I am heading to the hospital (that's what I tell him anyway), on account of I have a fractured back or something. He's very sympathetic. I have loaded up with painkillers and cough drops. I've never had one of these imaging scans before but I know you're supposed to lie relatively still and not be thrashing around in a coughing fit.

So quiet in there. Is it because it's so early or the narthex nature of the place? Quiet as a church. This is really it. The serious stuff. This is no turn your head and cough. I'm pretty sedated from the Darvocet, but not so much as to keep from wondering how I'd feel if I wasn't sedated. Does this make sense? First time for everything...something I'm going to be saying a lot of.

Clothes off, gown on, tech talk: no metal, no pacemaker, and so forth. I explain about my back, how I don't know that I can lie still for an hour, or that I can even lie down. The techs are beyond understanding, and it begins to penetrate my shell, my obliviousness, that I am not exactly the first person to enter the MRI clinic with a bad back, or an ache or pain of some sort.

I tell them about my cough, about how I won't be able to keep still without a cough drop clamped in my mouth, and will they allow that, and they tell me they will, no problem.

Okay, here comes the hard part: lying down. I'm in the room where the device is, and I sit on the sliding pallet, where two operating technicians let me lean into them, and very slowly they lower me to the pallet, onto my right side, from which position I can slowly roll onto my back. Somebody's thoughtful enough to put a pillow under my knees, which helps take some of the pressure off my lower spine.

I've got a major cough drop clamped in my molars, the back of my head, primed to dissolve and drip down my throat (soothe, coat and relieve, to coin a phrase), while I pray not to cough and a) completely ruin the testing process and b) wrench my spine again. The whole thing seems beyond dreamlike; I realize it is less than 24 hours since my episode at the chiropractor and things seem to be moving quickly and slowly at once. For a sick guy I seem to be doing quite a lot, moving around quite a bit.

The show's on the road. This is really it—sick stuff, anxiety stuff, all the stuff nobody wants to think about: sliding into the MRI device. Magnetic Resonance Imaging. If there was music piped in, I don't remember that. What I do recall is the tech, way out there in the beyond in her control booth, talking to me through a relay system, speakers inset in the tube, her voice cracking with all the hi-tech definition of a fast-food drive-thru window. She begins to explain the tests, the fact that this will be a series of tests, that she'll announce them as she goes, their sequence and length. "I'm starting the first test now, this will take about three and a half minutes." I'm all a-quiver.

Instantly I'm submerged in an electronic racket, what sounds like an Aphex Twin out-take skipping in my CD player, right in my ear. Or if that musical reference is no good, then: sounds like a dozen hard drives crashing all at once, and not very rhythmically either.

Only here's the significant thing: I almost fall asleep. Even with this beyond-Pluto solar pulse screeching in my ear, and my tensed up back, and the cough drop lodged in my molars a constant reminder of what might happen, still I manage to almost relax and drift into sleep. Must be those extra painkillers. The cough drop does its job, soothes coats relieves. I am lying down. The people around me seem to know what they're doing. The nonstop electronic racket is pretty easy to get used to, it turns out, like a summer thunderstorm at night. Anyway, when you haven't slept for a couple of nights, you'd be surprised where and when you can get some shut-eye.

So, it's noisy but not as bad as you think, going into this chamber. The Doughnut of Death. The fears: I'll have to go to the bathroom. I'll wet myself or worse. I haven't learned yet the concretizing effect of painkillers on the bowels, and the advantages to be derived therefrom. So, all in all, my first go-round in the MRI-go-round is, on the whole, almost on the relaxing side. "See, that wasn't so bad."

So when they slide me out like a finished loaf of bread, I find out what the real difficulty is: sitting up. I make a bit of a stab at it, struggling to rise from the pallet, but nothing doing. It's my vertebrae that are making a stab at me. The main technician and an assistant come over to help me up. Only then, again, do I think how these saints must be used to this sort of thing by now, people with tragic backs and other epic aches and twists, and again it begins to sink in on me that I am not exactly the only person in the world with physical complaints. That if I have now crossed some border into the land of Serious Hurt, it is also to have learned, to have it penetrate my noggin, that there is a land of Serious Hurt, that large numbers of people are suffering.

They are always suffering, and even though their exact population and citizenship, the members of the set may vary over time, they are always there. I am beginning to realize what thoughtful people always know, that there is a world of hurt. The thing I've always pushed out of mind. That the question is not: Why is this happening to me? but Why is this happening to so many millions of people?

So, it takes two people to raise me up to a sitting position, and it hurts like fuck when they do. As in an inescapable utterance of: *Owwwwwwwwwww!*

I rate sympathetic looks, they watch me, attend me, as I slide my butt over the edge, my bare feet to the floor.

Very slowly I dress myself again, and by the time I'm through, the wonderful tech has my MRI films ready for me in an envelope. Now that's service. Hope she wasn't expecting a tip. For some reason I still don't precisely understand, I resist the urge to examine the films. To be exact, there is no urge to examine the films. I take a peek into the el giganto envelope, just to make sure the films are really there. I see the wispy ghostly patterns and outlines of what appears to be somebody's body, and that's enough for me. MRI films are more disturbing than x-rays: they're like looking at my own autopsy, me as a selection of ghost-blue cold cuts.

So okay. My doctor's offices are up the street, just a couple of blocks, and even I can manage that on foot.

Chapter Five

THE PRONOUNCEMENT

I T'S STILL EARLY AS I shuffle down the block to my doctor's office, MRI films tucked under my arm. Some sort of hush. People seem to have gotten a jump on the holidays, perhaps. Not much traffic. In the doctor's offices things seem pretty calm. It's a Thursday morning one week before Christmas. Everyone is very nice and accommodating, nobody seems stressed. I explain my situation to the receptionist, how my doctor is out of the office but I absolutely need to get results of the tests he ordered, if they are available. Before long a nurse comes out to talk to me about all this and promises me an appointment with a doctor in about two hours. He'll go over my tests with me. Okay great. All I have to do is kill the next two hours.

As I recall this was, curiously, not too much of an agonizing suspenseful period of time. I know they make movies about just this sort of situation, but for some reason I wasn't too extraordinarily anxious, which is uncharacteristic for me. Was it because I thought there really was nothing more I could do? That I had after all even made it through the MRI, the thing I'd dreaded most, so what could be worse? Was it just a matter of the painkillers really doing their stuff? Or did I already know on some level what the results were bound to be?

Anyway, I didn't feel like sitting the waiting room (or waiting in the sitting room) for two whole hours, so I even went out, walked the three blocks to the Bourse Building on Fifth, had some coffee. It'd be pretty funny if I fell asleep in the middle of my life-altering doctor's appointment. Yes sir, just passing the time of day. I recall talking to Margot on my cellphone. Who called who? Does it matter? She satisfies herself that I made it in one piece through the MRI and wouldl get a doctor to look at me and tell me something. "Call me as soon as you hear," and so forth.

Time flies when you're having cancer. I shuffle on back to the doctor's office, and this time a nurse weighs me and shows me to a consultation room. Before long a doctor I've never seen before, Dr. Z.—Dr. Understudy—introduces himself and is about to start going over the results with me when he notices the results are not in. They're not in my file. The good doctor appears more disgusted than I am with this, and he leaves the room to round up those copies and find out what the hell's going on. So, there I am all alone again in the consult room, twiddling my thumbs, trying not to move too much. Sitting and sitting, doo doo doo.

The door remains closed. After a while I hear a single faint thwack on the outer wood, as if a large cat had scratched once to be let in, and promptly died. My curiosity, as they say, is aroused. I open the door, and in the plastic rack affixed upon it at approximate eye level I find not only my file but a several-page copy of what even I immediately understand are my blood and urine results, right where some nurse just dropped them. I look up and down the hall. Dr. Understudy is not in sight. Nobody is. It's like the Pentagon Papers just fell into my lap.

I take the results into the room and start to read them. Guess what: you don't have to have a medical degree from Harvard to figure these things out, especially when you have some idea of what to look for.

I put the papers back in the door rack, close the door again and wait for the doctor to return. I don't even think it's particular funny or noteworthy that I'd managed to see the results before he did. I don't remember thinking anything at all, or feeling any emotion beyond general disgust. Like I knew I was going to step in shit and I did. Like *What else is new?* Eventually the door opened.

I have been asked more than once what it was like to hear a doctor give me the diagnosis, one of those scenes that must rank in the top ten, maybe even the top five, of Events You Never Want to Have

Happen to You Or Even Think About Too Much. So, to answer that query once and for all, I give you, as honestly as I can recollect it, the following drama:

THE PRONOUNCEMENT (a play in one scene)

Curtain up. Medical examination room. White male, early to mid-40s, seated on examination table fully clothed: hiking boots, worn jeans, flannel shirt. Appearance of exhaustion: uncombed hair, sunken eyes, severely hunched-over.

Enter doctor with medical file and other papers. White male, late 40s: white coat, receding hairline, grim expression. Patient looks up, sees papers in doctor's hand.

PATIENT

(Glumly) I peeked already.

DOCTOR

(Reluctantly) Do you know what this means?

PATIENT

Yeah. I've got myeloma.

DOCTOR

(As if reassessing his first impression of patient) Are you a doctor?

PATIENT

No. My sister works at Fox Chase Cancer Center. I've been talking to her since this whole thing started. She told me what to look for in the tests. (Pause.) It is cancer, isn't it?

DOCTOR

Yes.

PATIENT

Shit.

Curtain (possibly plural). Previews to begin next Friday and run through the end of the following week. Opening night 6/6/06. Advance tickets are available for purchase through our theater website at any time, or by phone or in person at our box office Tuesdays through Fridays, 10 AM – 5 PM. Please remember: all sales are really, really final.

***

I THOUGHT THE DOCTOR WAS A jerk at first, but the fact is he was truly quite nice and helpful. I realize now how awful this must have been for him—having to give the diagnosis to a total stranger, a patient not one of his own, one he'd never seen until he'd walked into that room. He seemed stiff at first but that wore off quickly. He answered everything.

"I've been seeing a chiropractor. I guess that's not going to do me any good anymore?"

"No, it won't," he said definitively.

He did everything my sister told me to tell him to do. Wrote out a prescription for two types of OxyContin, the 12 hour time lapse (20 mg) and the breakthrough (5 mg). I remember stepping into the hall and phoning my sister, getting her office fax number, the doctor promptly setting off to fax my records over. There was nothing to do but get the work done. Perhaps I was in something of a state of shock. "Come on, there must be some mistake...I know I'm sick, but *cancer*?"

And there was this, too: a perverse sense of relief, as in: Now they'll take me seriously! (Famous tombstone: *I told you I was sick*).

Let's see, what else did I do on that lovely day? Low gray sky. The streets seemed emptier but I guess that was just me. Sitting in the Bourse in the AM, no tourists that I recall, but I kind of liked it that way. Last man on Earth. La Jettée. That abandoned-city aura. I hope you understand how this suited my mood. I didn't really want to be around people, crowds of happy active people. This is disease, the onset of disease, this is the worst of disease: the withdrawal, the wounded animalness, the retreat, the bitterness.

Let's see, what else did I do? Must've been distracted, a little screwy, cause here's what I did with doctor's OxyContin prescription: went to the pharmacy closest to my doctor's offices, Thomas Jefferson University Hospital, and gave them the prescriptions. Then I refused to stick around when they told me it might be an hour's wait to fill and decided to head for home, though this only meant having to make the return trip later that day or sometime the next. So, this contradictory rationale: I need to get the prescription filled right away...but no hurry picking it up, I already have some painkillers.

Also: standing in line, my cell phone goes off, and hey—it's the younger sister, Judith, calling because I'd spoken to her husband earlier in the week about the possible diagnosis. She's calling to check, with sterling timing, there in the line at the pharmacy. This kicks off a sort of Abbott and Costello routine—or no, more like a mob-related routine, with one of us trying to get information and the other attempting to convey it without giving anything away to eavesdropping strangers.

"So, where are you?"

"I'm in line at the pharmacy."

"And?"

"And here I am."

"Did you see the doctor?"

It becomes clear that my younger sister has been talking to her husband, but not to our mutual older sister.

"What do you know?"

"What Lou told me." That's her husband.

"And what did he tell you?"

I'm not being so circumspect because I'm a sadist, but because I'm very much in public, here in the line at the pharmacy. If I'd been on my way home, I wouldn't have been caught in a line when the call came, and there's a limit to what I want overheard. But also because I think it would be more sadistic to say: I can't talk now, I'll have to call you back.

She tells me what I told him.

"Yes, that's right," I say.

"And so, what's happened?"

"So, I had my appointment today, my test results came back."

It is patently obvious that people in line are listening. I know exactly what they're thinking. No, people, it's not *that*.

"And?"

"And I've got it. The results were positive."

I don't want to say "cancer." I don't want to say "myeloma." I know damn well what the people overhearing me are thinking... but I don't know if I give a damn anymore.

So we continue this sort of low-level mobster-style conversation.

"So what happens now?"

"It's already happening."

"But what do you do?"

"It's being done."

An elephant rounds a corner from the main hospital lobby, enters the pharmacy and settles itself in the room, close to the counter. I choose not to mention this.

"I'm at the pharmacy," I continue. "Getting my prescription filled. So, step number one, straight out the gate, getting my new prescription filled. I'm right on top of things."

"But what can I do?"

"Oh, don't worry about that."

"Joshua, what can I do?"

"You're doing it. Just by calling me you're doing it." The elephant puffs air through its snout, an emphatic exhalation just shy of snorting.

"Well, but what are you doing now?"

"I'm at the pharmacy. Nothing to it. Just getting some of my prescriptions filled here. That's all. Then off I go."

There's a woman standing in front of me, not doing a grand job of pretending not to listen, but it's not like someone auditioned her ahead of time. I appreciate her effort.

"Joshua, I'm trying to talk to you. You have cancer now, right?"

"That's about right, yes."

"Well, what can they... what are they going.... when do you start...?"

"It's okay, it's okay. Whoa, I'm practically at the counter. I'll call you later with more. You can call Margot."

"But what about Mom and Dad? Has anybody talked to Mom and Dad? Have you?"

"I haven't called them yet. Nobody's told them anything."

"So who's going to?"

"I'll tell them. Later today I'll call them. That will be me."

It's still December 15, 2005.

What's left for me that day? Cab home. An afternoon of phone calls. Friends. Two women in particular with whom I'd been pen-palling over the Internet. One is in New York State just north of the city; the other is a professor and poet about 100 miles west of me in Pennsylvania. They're both perfectly hushed and kind and say the most supportive things, and so I feel even worse that I haven't mentioned either to the other. I feel terrible not so much for what's been told to me but for what I now have to tell other people. I keep putting off my parents and putting them off. I call work, first the office manager (whose father died of cancer the previous year) and her quiet gasps and long groping silences are terrible. Terrible for both of us. I'm alone in my apartment, the overcast sky has turned dark, there is sleet and the sidewalks have gone slippery.

Just the thing for a paperboned cancer patient.

I leave a voicemail for my boss, the dean of the school, and she calls back promptly and is the soul of understanding. Her father, I will learn later, is in a losing battle with liver cancer. As I've said, she's a doctor, and everything she says is kind and projects hope about how myeloma is so much better understood now than ever, that it can be maintained and managed, and most of all that there is no limit to what she and the school will do to help me through this.

I'm thinking: *through* this?

There remain only my parents.

***

*W*HAT DID I DO THAT Friday? I took that Friday off. Now I remember. Stayed at home waiting to hear if I needed to go to Fox Chase... Waited to hear from Margot who had my files at Fox Chase. A series of embarrassing phone calls to friends and former girlfriends about a possible emergency ride to Fox Chase.

I do get a little bit of good news. Margot calls to say that the specialist, after looking at my records, didn't think my case was THAT bad. We could wait till Tuesday for an appointment, and meanwhile I should just keep taking painkillers. The phonecalls. Burning up the Internet, looking for data and stats on myeloma. Not good. Margot tells me to get a laxative to counteract the oxyconstipation.

What did I do that night? Don't remember. Is this when I began sleeping on the sofa? I made arrangements to have dinner Saturday out on Main Line with our parents and Judith's family. Judith and Lou come around to pick me up. They have been at the BodyWorlds exhibit at Franklin Institute, the dead people exhibit. They pick me up at my apartment give me a ride out to their house. Mom and Dad are there. There's an extended awkward moment. Nobody wants to seem too supportive, as that means acknowledging the elephant (or the crab) in the room.

Fractious as my relations with my immediate family have been, still there's the comfort of us being all there together. In a room together, I mean, looking each other in the eye or at least making a good effort at doing so. It helps. It's not as bad as when talking about it over the phone, that weird dislocation, like *Here I am giving you bad news but I'm not here really.* And the recipient of the news feeling worse because there's nothing they can do at the time BUT listen. So, a bit of safety in numbers. Being together with your kind.

We go out to the big fat Italian restaurant in Narberth. The restaurant is fine but it's really sinking in that I have no appetite. I order spaghetti and meatballs and the portions are generous but it sits there in front of me. It's not that I'm nauseated, it's that I simply have no appetite. It's the mood, the painkillers...as I recall the evening, it wasn't a total despondent washout. There was that indication that, since Fox Chase hadn't rushed me in, maybe things wouldn't be so bad. We'd gotten bad news, but perhaps in time, and I was in line to get the best treatment locally available.

Make no mistake, I've had all sorts of lucky breaks here. I live in a city with a crushing load of social problems but a commendable number of places to get good healthcare, assuming you've got the coverage. I can walk to a decent hospital. I can take an affordable cab ride to an esteemed myeloma specialist across town. I've got friends and family here.

Lots of people don't have that access and support and can't get specialized care, or even the correct diagnosis. I hear of cases all the time on the myeloma listserv of folks in isolated areas, remote, rural, where general practitioners are not up to date on rare blood cancers. Patients go months or years without a diagnosis, and then have trouble locating appropriate care and finding a way to get to it regularly. People uprooted. People having to move. I'll say it again: I'm lucky.

I'm tired and order a Pepsi for the caffeine, and my mother nags me about how it's not good for me. I have them wrap up my uneaten dinner in a doggy bag, which will follow me like a dog itself.

On the way back to my sister's, near-humiliation. Tell me to take a laxative, eh? I beg my sister to step on the gas and we reach her home in time, disaster narrowly averted. But the feeling sinks in: is this what I have to look forward to? Not two days post-diagnosis and already I've almost shit my pants. Note to self: lay off laxative.

The big idea is I'm going to spend the night with my younger sister's family, then get a ride with them to Bucks County the next day for the family Hanukkah get-together. I had managed presents for my older nephews but none for my niece and youngest nephew (Judith's children), having been a little distracted. But my mom got presents for them, wrapped them for me, made the presents look like they're from me.

I remember this night. My sister loaned me her portable CD player and I brought some discs with me. This is the night I took double the dose of OxyContin, maybe because my back began to hurt a little extra or maybe because I wanted to get a handle on that diarrhea. But I remember laying out on the guest bed and having a great fuzzy wave of warm come over me, as Volume 1 of Zappa's *You Can't Do That On Stage Anymore* revved around manically. The music had never sounded so good, that good. And I coasted off and everything was so good.

The next morning is dark with clouds. I go out for a walk with my sister's family very slowly, my arms out for balance. Overcast, gray. I am determined no to overdo the painkillers. By mid-day I am sitting in their dining room, by the bay window, scribbling madly in my journal. "Last thoughts, etc." Planning my funeral, setting things right. Making notes for my will. Well, you have to do it. Also sitting by myself as I'm embarrassed by ripping farts. I really am constipated. Horrible nonstop grandmotherly reeking farts.

The long ride from county to county to my older sister's. Hanukkah. Presents. Refusing to take my painkiller till the allotted time. I make a vow (a foolish one, it turns out) to stick to a strict schedule of painkiller meds. Regardless of how I may be feeling, I tell myself, I won't take any OxyContin beyond a strictly allotted dose at the same time every day: 20 mg upon waking, 20 mg at 6 PM. No matter what I'm feeling,

I will wait until the allotted time and I will take no more than that one pill. I'm wary of how much I enjoyed myself the previous night.

In privacy, plans are made between my older sister and me. How I'll arrive the following evening, spend the night, get a ride into the Cancer Center with her. Then I'll get a ride back into town with my younger sister and her family. After the discussion they take me home. It's dark and rainy on I-95 but brother-in-law #2 is a good driver. I get into my apartment just in time to avoid a mammoth painkiller-compacted bowel movement in my trousers. Welcome to the new normal.

It's Sunday, December 18, 2005, just past 8:45 PM. I'm losing sight of the basics: how to eat, sleep, dress. How to pack for an overnight stay. But that last is something I've got to do. Big day ahead of me tomorrow. Better get started now, what with me moving so slowly with the broken back and all, what with the head full of opiates. I scratch the head. Everything takes twice as long as usual. My travel bag is on the sofa. What needs to go in there, now?

I start with the little white bottle of Motrin, just in case. I don't want to leave it behind in my apartment. I don't want it to get lonely.

What was a spine being now a worm-eaten mast, what were ribs are rotted spars, and a storm is up inside of me, the failing boards are creaking, the warped planks protesting, the wind is up and the ship can't last and I can't remember if I even slept?

Chapter Six

MYELOMA, THE THING ITSELF

AH MYELOMA, THE POOR RELATION of the blood cancers.
Sometimes it feels as if my life has been nothing else but an arrangement for me to write that sentence.

Also known, at various times and places around our globe, as multiple myeloma, plasma cell myeloma, Kahler's disease, or Rustizky's disease. Similar to, but not nearly as well-publicized nor (at least until fairly recent times) as well-attended to by the medical world as other members of the hematologic cancer family, such as leukemia and lymphoma and their various sub-categories.

Those stuck-up bastards. I'll never forget the miserable Thanksgiving dinner I had at the Leukemias' house last year. What snobs! The way they looked at me when I asked for seconds, them and their shitty kids!

For example: wherever I have typed it into this ongoing Microsoft Word 2002 document on my graying laptop, the word "myeloma" appears with a squiggly red underline—the squiggly red Microsoft underline that means "what the hell is this word that you've properly misspelled?" (Suggested corrections from the software: *mycelia. Yeoman. Milkman. Melinda. My Loma.*) Does leukemia get the red underline? No. Does lymphoma? It does not. Only myeloma, and I refuse to apply the

"Add to Dictionary" or "Ignore All" functions that Microsoft provides. Let myeloma be the scarlet letters. Let The Big Red Squiggly One flourish throughout this computer file.

If this memoir accomplishes anything, let it be the abolition of that fuckingly mocking underline from beneath the noun in question from all future versions of Microsoft Word. (Note: As of January 2008, no dice: the condition persists in both Word 2003 and 2007 for Vista).

But things are taking a better, more public turn. Network news accounts have featured myeloma and its incidence in the population, in reports featuring the football player Elijah Alexander and former congresswoman and Vice Presidential candidate Geraldine Ferraro. Ferraro first spoke publicly about her 1998 diagnosis during her brave testimony to a Senate subcommittee meeting on blood cancers in summer 2001, one of the prominent patients to put a face to the disease. A 2008 New Yorker article focused on the Multiple Myeloma Research Foundation (MMRF) and its founder Kathy Giusti's goal of using business models to target effective treatments and possible cures for myeloma and to coordinate the research of related medical organizations.

So let us examine this disease, and firstly by name. What is its etymology? What does myeloma even mean, and why is it multiple?

Myelo-, from the Greek *myelos*, means "marrow," while -oma, a suffix derived from the Greek *karkinoma*, refers to our buddy the crab, or "cancer." That wasn't too hard: myeloma is a cancer of the bone marrow. (Oh myelolita, I have only words to play with...)

How does a cancer of the bone marrow begin, how does it spread, what, at the cellular level, does it do to your body?

What, you're asking me? Folks, you're really in trouble....

Let's take a look:

Blood cells begin, as all cells begin, as a stem cell. The term has unfortunately acquired "hot potato" political aura, but there is really nothing to it. A stem cell is simply a new and undifferentiated cell created in one spot or another in your body, before it has become a specialized cell (brain, nerve, blood), fully active and able to perform a particular function. Your body generates its blood stem cells (hematopoetic cells) in the marrow of your "long bones": the ribs, femur, humerus, pelvis and so forth.

From its origins as a stem cell, a blood cell may become one of the following: a red cell, a platelet, or one of the white cells or leukocytes. Leukocytes include T cells, NK cells (stands for Natural Killer, believe it or not), and B cells. Red cells carry oxygen. Platelets assist in clotting (sometimes too well). T and NK cells take part in cell-mediated immunity, which is he branch of the immune system that does not rely upon antibodies. The age of AIDS introduced us to T cells, and the types of infections that result when they malfunction—protozoal infections such as toxoplasmosis and *Pneumocystis* pneumonia, tuberculosis, and fungal infections. These types of pathogens multiply inside host cells and are killed when the infected cell is engulfed by a T cell.

In contrast to cell-mediated immunity is the so-called "humoral immunity," which results from the generation of antibodies to invading pathogens. Humoral immunity protects against pathogens that multiply outside the host cells, such as common viruses that cause colds and flu. According to the classic textbook *Molecular Biology of the Cell*, "Vertebrates inevitably die of infection if they are unable to make antibodies." Each antibody is made by a single type of terminally differentiated B cell called a "plasma cell" or an "effector B cell." In a healthy immune system there are billions of forms of antibodies, collectively called immunoglobulins, making up 20% of all protein found in blood serum. There are so many kinds that they are known in general as "polyclonal proteins."

All of the blood cells—red, white, and platelets—play an extremely important role in maintaining the good health too many of us take for granted. But when something goes askew in the development of those cells, when some malignancy enters and commandeers the process, we then have a blood cancer, a hematologic cancer.

What do you know, "hematologic" earns the red undersquiggle of suspicion from MS Word as well. Hey, Microsoft, what the fuck is your problem?

Put in the simplest terms, if something goes wrong early on in the process of blood cell formation, you will develop leukemia in some form. This is why leukemia is not uncommonly diagnosed in children.

If you make it past that, but then have problems with your lymphoid cells, you will then have the pleasure of contracting some flavor of lymphoma. If you've managed to dodge those bullets, but screw up towards the end of the process, where the plasma cells are differentiated—then, you lucky devil, you will have myeloma. This is why myeloma patients on average skew towards the elderly, at least 50 years of age and older, because it's the last thing that can go wrong in the stages of blood cell development. Also unknown is why the disease, at least according to records of North American patients, appears in significantly higher numbers in black patients than whites.

In a process which remains mysterious, in myeloma the plasma cells go haywire. Instead of making a rich variety, the bone marrow begins to produce one type of plasma cell with some abnormal fragment of an antibody in runaway abundance. So many uncontrolled copies of this abnormal single protein are generated that it will be known as the "monoclonal protein." Its overabundance will be seen in blood and urine tests, and its telltale presence is exhibited as a sharply elevated spike in the results of an SPEP (serum protein electrophoresis) and/or UPEP (urine protein electrophoresis) test. That spike is the "M-spike" that one begins promptly to hear so much about when diagnosed: not M for myeloma but M for monoclonal. It's also called "paraprotein."

About 3% of people over 50 and 5% of people over 70 have raised levels of paraprotein. This is a benign condition called monoclonal gammopathy of unknown significance (MGUS). MGUS doesn't cause any symptoms but carries a slight risk of progression to myeloma (about 1% per year).

The condition beccomes myeloma when organs and tissues begin to be impaired by proliferating plasma cells and high levels of para-protein. It's not bad enough having these cells in abundance; they also serve to crowd out the other plasma cells you should be creating. And not only the plasma cells but the other blood cells too, the other whites (the Ts and the NKs), and even our friends the reds. You have mutant blood.

Mutant blood: sorry to report that mutation at the blood cellular level does NOT result in the ability to turn invisible, swing from the tops of skyscrapers via spiderwebs, or shoot laser beams from the eyes with or without pinpoint accuracy. Mutant blood cells, myeloma cells, will fuck you up proper and eventually kill you. Let us count the ways.

In 1975, Durie and Salmon published a staging system for myeloma based upon four major symptoms which a patient may present. Any one of these is an indication of myeloma, and in combination they make it a lead pipe cinch to diagnose. The four are: Elevated calcium levels in blood (C); renal dysfunction (R); anemia (A); bone damage (B). That's right, the acronym for this set of symptoms is CRAB. As in cancer the crab. Should anyone complain about my sick sense of humor, I direct you to the sick bastard who coined the acronym.

Let's examine the mechanics of myeloma's symptoms, and precisely how it goes about its nasty business. First, bone damage. Normally, your body contains cells related to bone production: these are osteoblasts and osteoclasts. Osteoblasts are responsible for the formation of new bone cells in your skeletal system, the routine regeneration of new bone tissue to replace the old. Osteoclasts handle the normal breakdown of older bone cells, part of the routine regeneration that occurs within our bodies all the time.

Now here's where myeloma really does its dirty work. Myeloma cells somehow (in a manner only recently beginning to be understood) stimulate osteoclast activity, so that bones are worn or eaten away at a much higher rate. At the same time, the osteoblast activity is reduced, if you will, so that worn out bone cells are not being replaced. So erosion of your bones is accelerated while renewal of bones is not. A medical degree is not required to see the problem here. A myeloma patient, regardless of age, will exhibit advanced osteoporosis and weakened bones. X-rays of bones will even display a moth-eaten appearance, with holes and frayed and "punched-out" areas. Pain from this condition is a constant, and fractures are common.

As if this wasn't enough, masses of plasma cells form tumors in the bones. These plasmacytomas look like a soft mass of red jelly and are lytic, meaning they cause lysis of bone. Because plasmacytomas are almost always in more than one spot in the skeleton upon diagnosis, the dieases earns the qualifier "multiple." The Durie-Salmon staging system counts these lesions as an estimate of tumor burden, but modern staging is usually based on more quantitative criteria.

Anemia: with all those excess plasma cells going to town in your marrow, your other cells will scarcely have room to breathe...and neither will you. Red blood cell production is compromised, which means less oxygen being delivered where it should be throughout your body. Concurrent with this, platelet production is often thrown off balance.

As an indication of just how bizarrely and idiosyncratically the disease manifests itself from patient to patient, some myeloma sufferers may find themselves with increased platelet counts and the concomitant risk of thrombosis from internal clots. Others will experience decreased platelet counts, and may find themselves popping mysteriously stubborn nosebleeds, sometimes while watching Sam Fuller movies.

Hypercalcemia: well, with all that bone deterioration going on, you wind up with excess amounts of calcium being released into bloodstream. You know how your mom told you to drink up your milk because calcium is good for you? Well, your Mom didn't know shit. Too much calcium in your blood causes a host of problems, especially fatigue, disorientation, and general bad emotional states. When it really goes overboard, you run into heart and kidney failure.

Renal dysfunction. Oh yeah, this is great, are we having fun yet? There's so much crud in your blood your kidneys can't filter it all. Elevated proteins, too much calcium...at some point your two kidneys are going to cry uncle. Many myeloma patients are diagnosed following sudden kidney failure. That must be fun—to experience kidney failure and then find out the reason for it is cancer. But kidney problems are something I've managed to avoid so far. Why? Who knows. Just lucky, I guess. This disease has generally known characteristics but is next to impossible to predict the course from one particular patient to another. Some patients will experience severe kidney problems from the treatment of the disease. You can't win.

****

Facing page. Blood cell lineages and related cancers. From a hematopoetic stem cell (hemocytobast), cells take either the myeloid lineage (not shown in detail) or the lymphoid lineage. Different types of blood cancers (indicated in bold) can occur at several stages during the maturation of the progenitor stem cells. Acute lymphoblastic leukemia (ALL) is an abnormal proliferation of lymphoblasts. Natural killer cells can give rise to a leukemia, though this is rare. Abnormal proliferation of mature lymphocytes results in lymphoma or in the inaccurately named "prolymphocytic" leukemia. Both T and B cells cause lymphomas; Hodgkin's disease is a type of B-cell lymphoma. Abnormal proliferation of the class of B cells called plasma cells causes myeloma.

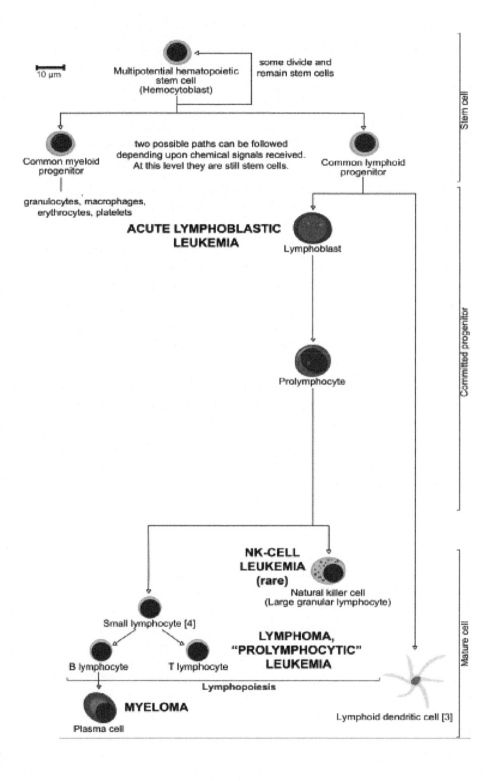

10 μm

Multipotential hematopoietic stem cell (Hemocytoblast)

some divide and remain stem cells

Stem cell

Common myeloid progenitor

two possible paths can be followed depending upon chemical signals received. At this level they are still stem cells.

Common lymphoid progenitor

granulocytes, macrophages, erythrocytes, platelets

ACUTE LYMPHOBLASTIC LEUKEMIA

Lymphoblast

Committed progenitor

Prolymphocyte

NK-CELL LEUKEMIA (rare)

Natural killer cell (Large granular lymphocyte)

Small lymphocyte [4]

LYMPHOMA, "PROLYMPHOCYTIC" LEUKEMIA

B lymphocyte

T lymphocyte

Lymphopoiesis

MYELOMA

Plasma cell

Lymphoid dendritic cell [3]

Mature cell

*W*E HAVE NOW EXAMINED, IN bitten-thumbnail form, where myeloma comes from and how it does its damage. You get that. But who saw it first? Who called it like it is and when? Some medical history is in order.

Thomas Alexander McBean, in September 1844, was an English grocer, 44 years of age, and already father to nine children. Way to go, Mr. McBean! While holidaying with his wife and two eldest children in the French countryside, he emerged with some energy from an underground cavern and "instantly felt as if something had snapped or given way within the chest, and for some minutes he lay in intense agony, unable to stir."

I can't tell you how miserable that description made me when I first read it. It was so familiar, but it also arrived a bit too late for me to tell that poor suffering devil how genuinely sorry I felt, and continue to feel, for him. Myelomics know exactly what you experienced, Thomas McBean, and more than a century and a half later, the only thing we can do is try to explain what was murdering you by pieces.

The episode of the cave was not without presage, though no one could possibly have understood the problem at the time. McBean's family had noted his fatigue and stooped posture during the previous year. That day he was finally able to hobble away from the site of his collapse, but a month later, having returned to England, he suffered another attack of debilitating bone pain. Treatment included bleeding by leeches "followed by considerable weakness for two or three months." Gee, you think?

Throughout 1845, McBean suffered further excruciating attacks, and by autumn of that year had constant sharp pain in the "chest, back, and loins," forcing him into a perpetually bent posture, only able to get into or out of bed by slow crawling "on all-fours." His urine was noticeably thick, "like pea soup" (I avoid the obvious pun). His treating physicians, William Macintyre and Thomas Watson, were so puzzled by this last symptom, and by further unusual qualities which the urine exhibited after a series of tests, that they sent a sample to a Dr. Henry Bence Jones.

Dr. Bence Jones was very interested indeed. Thirty-one years of age in 1845, he was already one of London's leading specialists in chemical pathology and kidney diseases in particular, and was well on his way to becoming one of the Empire's most prominent physicians. His patients would include Charles Darwin, Thomas Huxley, and Michael Faraday, and he later became a friend and colleague of Florence Nightingale.

In November 1845, Bence Jones re-performed some of the heating and chemical tests that McBean's GPs had made and was struck by what he termed the "animal matter," or protein, so persistently and abundantly evident in the urine. According to his own tests, McBean was excreting the phenomenal amount of over 60 grams per day of the substance, which he termed "hydrated deutoxide of albumen."

Bence Jones paid a house call to the patient on November 15. McBean, while managing some intervals of brief recovery and strength, remained overall in dreadful condition, having developed a deep cough and diarrhea in addition to his almost constant physical agony. The case was hopeless. Despite treatment with alum (recommended by Bence Jones), along with opium and morphine, McBean died on New Year's Day, 1846.

An autopsy revealed the appalling damage done to McBean's skeleton, particularly those areas where he had experienced the most pain: "...the ribs, which crumbled under the heel of the scalpel, were soft, brittle, readily broken, and easily cut by the knife. Their interior was filled with a soft 'gelatiniform substance of a blood-red colour and unctuous feel.' (Unctuous marrow. Good title for a book). The sternum was also involved...[T]he thoracic and lumber vertebrae had the same changes as found in the ribs and sternum...."

Of great interest are the details noted by surgeon John Dalrymple of the Royal Ophthalmic Hospital, who closely examined McBean's ribs and vertebrae during the autopsy. He saw how the disease clearly began *within* the bones, where the marrow had first mutated before spreading to produce numerous "round, dark-red projections" visible through holes eaten through the bones. Dalrymple placed samples of the transformed marrow under a microscope and found them composed almost entirely of oddly massive cells, most of them up to twice as large as a normal blood cell, with enlarged and even doubled nuclei. The engravings Dalrymple made of these cells match the appearance of what are known today to be myeloma cells.

At the time, no one saw this peculiar case in terms of cancer, blood or otherwise. It was described instead as an extreme case of mollities ossium (softening of the bones), instances of which had of course been diagnosed previously in other patients without any idea being formed of the cause. But significant evidence was being accumulated, even if the context into which to place it had not yet been conceived. And it was Dr. Bence Jones who made the critical bad-marrow/high-protein connection. In his accounts of McBean's case (*Lancet*, 1847-48), he wrote "I need hardly remark on the importance of seeking for this oxide of albumen in other cases of mollities ossium."

It is this insight for which Bence Jones is chiefly remembered today, more than the famous patients in his lifetime, more than his career-long studies of diabetes and kidney disease. In fact, at time of his death in 1873, there appeared no particular interest in this particular discovery in the area of microscopic urine analysis. But fear not. Decades later, "Bence Jones protein" is the fingerprint, a high-water mark, if you will, of myeloma diagnosis, its presence a major tell-tale sign of the disease. Immortality is yours, Doctor Bence Jones! The history of your name has been written in urine!

Thomas McBean stands as the first recorded case of multiple myeloma. Emphasis on the word "recorded," from a retrospective point of view, as the disease had not yet been named—that would take another three decades.

Of course evidence exists of similar medical cases previous to McBean's. (What did David Bowie say? It's not who does it first, it's who does it second?) There is the dreadful case of Sarah Newbury, who died in London in 1844, aged only 39, four years after beginning to display pronounced symptoms of fatigue and severe back pain. One night in 1842, intending to assist her, Newbury's husband lifted her to carry her to bed; beneath his hands, she felt "as if her thighs were being broken into a thousand pieces," as they essentially were, and she never walked again. Her bones, particularly the femurs and sternum, displayed in autopsy the same moth-eaten texture as did McBean's two years later, as well as the same morbidly gelatinous marrow. Unfortunately, there is no record of any analysis made of Newbury's blood or urine, but presumably the fatal proteinuria would have been found, as her case has all the hallmarks of myeloma.

Great Britain being in the mid-19th century the most industrially advanced nation on the globe, it is no surprise to discover its physicians at the forefront of recording unusual new diseases. There is also an additional footnote. Note the ages of the patients mentioned here. Newbury, 39. McBean, 45. Of course life expectancies were shorter then, but those are still very young ages at which to contract myeloma. Given that industrial/environmental factors are often cited as probable cause for the disease, could England's status as the leading industrial nation possibly have some connection to the relatively youthful nature of its first myeloma patients? Or is it simply that the most technically advanced nation of its era had the resources and professionals well-educated enough to notice this peculiar ailment?

But of course myeloma was also being noticed elsewhere in the world. German physician Hermann Weber noted in 1867 a 40-year-old patient (again, curiously young) presenting with constant severe back pain and chronic head colds, who died just months later. Autopsy revealed bones full of our friend the red jelly.

Wilhelm Friedrich Kühne—a noted German physiologist who coined the word "enzyme," from the Greek "to leaven"—also described a case. While working as professor of physiology in Amsterdam in 1868 saw a patient (40 years old! Again!) "unable to lie on his back...with trouble sleeping because of pain and curvature of the spine." The patient died nine months after first appearing with symptoms. No slouch, Kühne examined the patient's urine and traced its suspicious cloudiness to the same protein levels as those discovered by Bence Jones twenty years before.

We now come to one of the most mysterious portions of this entire affair, the case of the Russian physician "von Rustizky." I have been unable to learn very much at all about this gentleman, not even his first name. The only indication we have is the initial "J." (Joshua? Not likely). Von Rustizky published a report in German in 1873, describing his autopsy of a 47-year-old (!) patient who had died from pronounced tumors within the skeleton. These tumors appeared to Rustizky as obviously carcinomic in origin (he was right), originating in the marrow of the bones and occurring in no less than eight spots in the patient—including various ribs, vertebrae and the right humerus. It was Rustizky who termed these numerous instances of marrow cancer "multiple myeloma." Reportedly, in Russia, "Rustizky's disease" is often the preferred term for the disease. Why more is not known about this physician I cannot comprehend.

Prague, 1889: Dr. Otto Kahler described the case of a fellow physician, Dr. Loos, who had succumbed two years previously (at age 46!) to all the symptoms of myeloma: severe skeletal crumbling (Loos suffered such severe damage to the spine as to become a dwarf), chronic bronchial infections and the same turbid urine, full of Bence Jones protein. Autopsy revealed the same mutant marrow composed of myelomatic cells. "The ribs were soft and could be broken with minimal effort." So classic was this case that Kahler became closely associated with the history of myeloma, which in some places—outside of Russia, apparently—is referred to as Kahler's disease. He was to perish of cancer himself, a malignancy of the tongue, shortly after his 44th birthday. (Did anybody live past their forties in those days?)

The first American case of myeloma was reported in 1894, the patient a Caucasian female aged 40(!). Meanwhile, x-rays and their potential use in medical diagnosis had recently been discovered, with a Dr F. P. Weber specifically noting their helpfulness in cases of myeloma. The general picture was coming into focus. By the beginning of the 20th century, x-rays were coming to be used in diagnosis. And as advances in science were linked to medicine, so did they come to be applied to the particular sub-type of cancer, most notably, if slowly, in the field of treatment. By 1928, the two doctors Geschickter and Copeland published findings based on an overview of every known or probable case of multiple myeloma reported since 1848, which by then numbered 425.

Do the math: that's fewer than six cases reported per year over 80 years. Of course, general medicine, not to mention the public, was not especially mindful of the disease nor its signposts during that period. Still, only 5.31 cases of myeloma per year? That can't be right. Today, in the US alone, more than 15,000 new cases are diagnosed annually. Most notably, Geschickter and Copeland worked up a list of six main symptoms of the disease: back pain; anemia; chronic renal disease; presence of Bence Jones protein; chronic skeletal fractures—what doctors like to call an SRE, Skeletal Related Event—and "multiple involvement of tumors of the skeletal trunk." The use of bone marrow biopsies began in the 1920s. Plasma/myeloma cells: to me they look like slices of deviled egg, like cross-sections of hardboiled eggs.

The disease was still rare, not particularly well known outside of rarefied medical study; its origins were and continue to remain mysterious. And, oh yeah, one more thing: while treatments have improved significantly since the early 1990s, there remains no effective cure as of this writing in 2017.

***

*U*NTIL ABOUT THE MID-1990S, A diagnosis of myeloma was effectively a death sentence. Some progress in treatment had been made, when the process of chemotherapy, successful in other cancers, was applied to the disease. The nitrogen mustard agent Melphalan in particular got some results. Nitrogen mustard is what it sounds like—a close relative of the gas used in chemical warfare in World War I.

And by results, I mean the patient's life was extended by an indeterminate, and not terribly long, period of time. There was and remains no cure. The disease remained poorly understood; it always was one of the rare ones.

But since then, the mid-1990s, there has been what appears to be a reversal on that account. Precisely because myeloma seemed such a hopeless dead-ended backwater of cancer research, some doctors seemed to find the field wide open.

There exists, at this time of writing, The Leukemia & Lymphoma Society. Is it the Leukemia, Lymphoma and Myeloma Society? It is not. Myeloma has to make its own societies: The International Myeloma Foundation. The Multiple Myeloma Research Foundation.

Is there a Blood Cancer Society, where we can all get along and share? Presently, no. Perhaps because of the term "blood cancer" itself, way up there on the repulse-o-meter. Who wants to hear of such a thing? It's like "saliva feces" or "pubic cankers." One imagines Dracula himself retching in disgust.

Please understand that I'm just kidding. When you have cancer, you have to make your laughs where you can. The Leukemia & Lymphoma Society is an outstanding organization; I've done fundraising for them, and a considerable amount of the Society's work is directed at fighting myeloma. No one is willfully ignoring or seeking to cover up information about the disease. All it is about is playing catch- up, which the medical world is certainly doing, particularly in the last ten years. It appears to have been misunderstood, even viewed as a condition of or corollary to old age rather than an actual cancer of its own. So what is it?

Increasing medical attention has been paid to myeloma, particularly in the past ten years, with a series of important clinical trials and applications of new drugs and/or new applications of established ones.

Which is what I hope to address here. Not my myeloma but all of them. By necessity I have to describe my case, the one I know in fullest detail, but I'm just the example. My subject is myeloma itself. The squiggly red underline. To renew our World War II metaphors here: The Thin Red Squiggly Underline.

I believe myeloma's cancer-come-lately status is due in large part to its having been perceived, until recently, as a disease of the elderly. As if it were part or a condition of old age itself, and what's the point in studying that? There appears the suggestion that myeloma was considered hopeless, especially in the elderly, and that once diagnosed, there was little point in extended treatment or seeking a cure. Diagnosis is often missed in older patients. A patient over the age of 65 presents with fatigue, aching bones, a sore back. "So what?" says the examining physician. "You're old!"

There is also the uncomfortable fact that myeloma, at least in the US, afflicts blacks twice as often as whites—and we all know how America pays closer attention to the problems of blacks than whites. (Personally, I have wondered why, in all my visits to and treatments at two various cancer centers did white patients so overwhelmingly outnumber blacks? Not that everyone I saw could possibly have been a myeloma patient, but still. Why, during my three-week hospital confinement for my stem cell transplant, did this same disparity appear to prevail on my floor?)

Ah, but the worm turns. Or the crab. Myeloma is increasingly seen in people under the age of 65. I was 44 at the time of my own diagnosis, and Caucasian. Nobody knows why this is, because nobody knows what causes myeloma in the first place, just as nobody knows an effective cure. But there have been remarkable advances over the past decade in research into the disease. With a variety of new medications and other treatments in current effective use, and with proven histories of patients surviving longer with the disease than ever before, a diagnosis of myeloma is now, I'm thrilled to say, more like a death paragraph. So, thanks to more and newer sorts of myeloma patients, it has begun to get the recognition it deserves.

It's not pretty. Fatigue, weakened bones, inability to get around much, to be very active, to hold down a job. It makes you elderly before your time, and if you are already elderly, it makes life even more difficult. Depending on the nature of their work, myeloma patients may find themselves unable to continue employment, which of course raises serious issues regarding health coverage. Do I have to mention the emotional toll, the psychological damage? Treatments such as chemotherapy, pharmaceuticals, and stem cell transplants, however beneficial, may take several months to complete, often have serious side effects, and frequently require extensive time off from work and career. Many people cannot afford that time. Even a relatively stable subject, in partial or "complete" remission, may find him- or herself simply too tired to do, or easily do, things that once came easily: travel, exercise, housework. It's tough, it's tough. Even with a great network of family and friends, it's tough, because it's tough on them. And this, of course, is not specific to myeloma but to all cancers, and major illnesses.

So my advice to you is to get cancer when you're young and healthy. That way you'll be best equipped to handle all the little difficulties and minor inconveniences which the disease may cause.

***

*W*HAT ARE THE STATISTICS FOR the survival of leukemia, lymphoma and myeloma?

Survival is measured in several ways, so it is important to define each measure. The survival statistics are often presented as five-year survival: that is, the percentage of people who survive five years from the date of diagnosis. The five-year survival rates for the blood cancers (for all age groups) are: leukemia, 48%; Hodgkin lymphoma, 85%; non-Hodgkin lymphoma, 60% and myeloma, 32.4%. Leukemia survival rates by type of disease (for all age groups) are: acute lymphoblastic leukemia (ALL), 64%; chronic lymphocytic leukemia (CLL), 74.2%; acute myeloid leukemia (AML), 19.8% and chronic myeloid leukemia (CML), 39.3%. These figures differ for children ages 0-19 and people over 75.

Oh, just great, so I've got a 2 in 3 chance of dying before 5 years.

How did I get this impression that myeloma is Cancer Lite? Turns out it's got the worst survival rate of the blood cancers. How can they do this to me? Five years, that's all I've got? Like Ziggy Stardust? I'm no better than Ziggy Stardust? So what, I'll just have enough time to maybe finish this book and see it into print? Maybe?

Better type fast.

Chapter Seven

FOX CHASE

O R CRAB CHASE WOULD BE more like it.

Is it part of the same day or is it part of the same night? I could never sleep through the night in a strange place, and this is the first time I've spent the night in my sister's house, with or without a crumbling spine. I start out on the front sofa...then the fireplace room couch...then the easy chair. The dogs. I hear my brother-in-law sneaking in from his job, the night shift, trying not to wake me, and I oblige him by not speaking, by not indicating that I am awake. I can *hear* him tiptoeing.

I haven't figured out the medications yet. I don't want to take the 12-hour OxyContin. 12 hours! I'll be a junky for sure. I don't want to live with the painkillers, I just want them to help me out a bit, like an annoying neighbor whose help you have to ask for sometimes—like for hauling out the trash, but you don't want the guy moving in with you.

So here comes dawn. The empty fishtank effect, the dry fishtank, me on the bottom. I've scarcely gotten undressed or unpacked so I'm ready to go when my sister comes down and starts the coffee.

"Did you sleep okay?"

Oh yeah. Like a baby.

"The painkillers helped you sleep, right? You're taking the 12-hour pills, right, like I told you?"

"Maybe."

"Maybe? What do you mean *maybe?* Do you want to feel better or not? Are you going to follow instructions or...look, you're going to have to learn to follow doctors' instructions now. You're a cancer patient now, Joshua, I'm really sorry but you're going to have start doing a lot of things that you never did before. Things that you won't like but you're going to have to do them."

"Yeah, I know, but...I'm afraid of...you know, getting a dependency."

"It's not a dependency if you're having pain. This is just getting started and you'll have to get used to taking medication the way it's prescribed. This is just getting started. Here, have some coffee."

I take one of the pills. I could start singing "The Needle and the Damage Done," but that would really be obnoxious, even for me.

We're both up so early. There's time for a shower, a shave. Fragments of human routine in the weak dawn. Outside it's very cold; I'm shuffling beside my sister, she's carrying my bag. I'm so fucked up. I really have no idea what to expect. The cold, the dawn. Drive me anywhere, I wouldn't know, wouldn't care. My back is a dull thump. Drive me to the airport, get me on a flight to the Caribbean, let me out, let me die.

Hhhaaaaaaaaaaaaaaaack, hack-hack-hack. My cough, cold, seriousness thereof.

Back down into the city. How do people live out here in these suburbs? Nice and open but I see no points of reference, no directional hints. Guess it takes a few years to figure it out. We halt at train tracks, listen to the news. Well, here we are. The sign says Fox Chase Cancer Center. I guess they're not kidding around. 7:30 AM, rise and whine. Well, it's official now.

Hanging out in the lobby. Actually I got put into the system the past Friday (over the phone, the day I was almost admitted on emergency basis, and I made those frantic phone calls. Remember?) so registering as a new patient doesn't take very long. What do I really remember of this? I see it in my head, fragments of it. I can prove I was there, but everything must have been distorted by sleeplessness, by drugs, by fear. I get a blue card, I get a wristband. My mom shows up. More on that later.

Down the hall. Am I the youngest person here? About looks that way. Certainly I don't see any children, which is fine with me, and I wonder if there is a special wing here for them. Yeah, I think I'm definitely the youngest. In future days I'll wonder, seeing people together, who is the patient and who is the "support" person.

Fireplace. Pale flames. There's a weird moment when I look up at the plate glass observation window and see the fireplace reflected over the drive outside, and I think I'm looking at a car in flames.

In we go: the consultation room. My sister comes along. Waiting and waiting, I'm too tired to be worried. I shuffle off for a leak. When I come back, here's my doctor, the big cheese himself. Dr. S, supposedly the best that family connections can finagle. He's got an assistant, too, a nurse practitioner named Brooke who works with my sister. They're all trying not to look too horrified as I cough and sneeze during this preliminary interview, because even I know how bad it is.

So after the preliminary bullshit patient-background questions we get down to the good stuff. They've got my records and test results, everybody knows what I've got, so they start telling me how they're going to treat it.

Radiation. Check. Is my hair going to fall out?

"Your hair's falling out already," says my sister.

I give her the finger.

Chemo?

"Well, probably not. We think we can get by on pills you take at home. Dexamethasone, for instance."

What's that?

"Steroids, for strength."

"Steroids, huh? For real, I'm going to be on steroids?"

"This is conventional," they tell me.

Great. Can't wait to beat Cal Ripken's record. I hadn't yet learned the difference between anabolic steroids, which bodybuilders use to get swole, and corticosteroids, which mess with your immune system and your mind.

"And Zometa. That's a bone-building chemical you'll get once a month in an infusion."

Ah ha! So there is chemotherapy.

"Well, no, it's only once a month, and the infusion only takes fifteen minutes."

Zometa, huh? All right, what else?

"Thalidomide."

What the fuck is this guy talking about? Thalidomide? The monster baby stuff? It's not enough I have cancer, now my cock is gonna fall off with monster babies? Uh, aren't there a few side effects associated with that?

"Well ah, heh heh, as a matter of fact there are. If you're planning on having children, you may want to contact a sperm bank in the near future."

Oh, I'm so glad my mom and sister are sitting in on this consultation. So now there's something else I have to schedule.

What I don't mention is that ever since I started the painkillers, my cock's had all the fighting power of a beached jellyfish. I mean, I haven't had hard-on in days. What am I supposed to do?

Okay, so all these fucking pills. What about them? What about my back? What are you going to do about that, genius? I got a spine like thin ice.

"Well, we don't do that here. You would see an orthopedic specialist. There are many things he might do. They might put balloons in your vertebrae and inflate them and ease some of your discomfort that way."

What the fuck is this guy talking about? Balloons in my fucking spine? And then what? Party favors and confetti? What the fuck is the matter is the matter with you? What are you talking about, balloons? Any other bright ideas?

"There are some procedures where they use cement to brace your spine."

Cement? They're going to cement my fucking spine?

"Well, not cement exactly. A cement-*like* substance."

Oh, well that's different. You had me worried there for a minute. But if it's only a cement-like substance....

"The thing is the timing. We won't be able to treat your cancer and your back at the same time. The treatment for one will preclude treatment for the other, thanks to blood-thinning and so on. So you have to make decisions, and pretty quickly."

Bottom line: I can't start the thalidomide (the main treatment) and then start treating my back in a possible operation. I have to see the back guy first, find out what he thinks, then begin thalidomide. But can't take too long, because I have to start taking the thalidomide ASAP, because, heh heh, we want to get started on fighting the cancer.

So, basically, it's a toss-up right now as to which horrible problem gets taken care of first. Plus, I have to masturbate and I can't.

"Wait. We haven't mentioned the bone marrow transplant yet."

"What bone marrow transplant?"

"If all goes according to plan, if you hold up under the medication, in about six months you should be able to have a bone marrow transplant. Of course you'll need to be typed for a marrow match. And you have to pick the right specialist to do it. We don't do it here."

***

I'M COUGHING AND SNEEZING. THE doctors have a look in their eyes like they don't like this one bit.

"How long have you been coughing like that?"

"Like what?" Hack hack hack!

"Like that."

"I dunno. Since I was diagnosed, I guess."

"What color's the sputum?"

Uh, you know, I haven't given that a whole lot of attention. Wasn't that a bestseller or something? Let's see what I can come up with.... Haaaaaack hack hack into a Kleenex. "Uh, it's yellow. You want to see it?"

"Uh, no, that's okay."

The NP is busy writing up a prscription for an antibiotic.

They're worried about the infection, but all I care about is the fact that every time I cough, it feels like somebody's kicking my spine, and I really think I might break another bone right there in front of everyone. In other words, I almost wish I would get infected and croak already and end all this bullshit.

The NP gives me a batch of prescriptions...antibiotics, dexamethasone. "This stuff is going to make your head spin."

Like it ain't already? I don't process that remark until much later. Gee, and it's only 11 AM. Quite a day. Accomplished so much already.

"I'll see you tomorrow for the biopsy," says Dr S.

You mean I gotta come back tomorrow? Oh yeah, great. Well, I'm really looking forward to that. So now what?

"We've got to get you over to radiation," Margot reminds me.

Off to another wing. Radiation has its own little environment. Like buried underground, if you know what I mean. We're talking Incredible Hulk time here. I'm tagging along after my sister like I'm her little brother or something. Can't I just lie down?

No. We have to get you into radiation. "It will target the areas in your spine where the myeloma is causing so much pain."

Funny how my sister seems to know so many of the people. It's almost as if she really does work here!

Next thing I know I'm in the radiation simulation room. Simulation, what the hell. My sister is explaining that before they bombard me with radiation, they have to do a test first. Like a dress rehearsal. I'm afraid the finer points of this are lost on me. I'm starting to crash.

"Take another pill," my sister says. "That's what it's for. Use it."

There's really only one thing that grabs my attention now. They've got me changed into a hospital gown (not easy, back flaring up), so I know something's up. Am I really sick or not? Uh oh, I knew this was coming. I'm going to have to lie down. Forget it.

I'm in the "simulation" room, which looks real enough to me, with a metal tray for me to lie on under some sort of mammoth panel. The technician is telling me I have to lie down and I'm telling them to forget it.

"You have to lie down."

"Then I can't get up."

"We'll help you up."

"How long do I have to lie here?"

Patiently (ha ha, you get it) the process is explained to me. They have to target the areas in my body that they radiate, using my MRI films for a guide. (Gee, you mean that thing is really good for something?) They'll save the targeted areas in the computer so their machines know where to hit me every time I come in for a treatment. In other words, an undress rehearsal. They don't want to hit the wrong spots when they radiate me for real. I don't want them to hit the wrong spots either.

I've got two techs working over me, marking x's and angles with green and black marker.

"Will that wash off?"

"Yes, but we have to tattoo you."

They're not kidding. So, finally, I'm going to get some tattoos. Out come the needles. Ow. Fuck. Why isn't that painkiller doing its job? This is not very artful, people. They're just sticking me with a needle and some black ink. Between the dots and the marker I look like some kindergartener's blueprint. Or like a bombadier's target screen: my cancerific bones being the target, I guess.

For a simulation, they're taking their sweet fucking time. I have the dim understanding that after this, I've got to put up with the real thing. That's right...

Here comes the worst part of all: having to get up off the fucking table. I'm helpless as a dead tuna. Two techs get my shoulders and ease me up into an upright position, the perfect posture to give my lower back a jolt. This will become very familiar over the next several days. In fact, this is what I will dread the most about the treatment: having to get on and off the table.

Recollection gets a little blurry here. At some point I get introduced to the doctor in charge of radiation treatment. It occurs to me to ask if he's a real doctor or only an ongoing part of the simulation, but I suppose this is not the time for Philip K. Dick references. Best not to poke fun at the doctor with the laser gun. He gives me the rundown: "Ten days of radiation. You may experience some pain. Don't be afraid to take the painkillers. You will be feeling better very soon. If not, let me know." He grips his left wrist with his right hand. Why? Does it hurt?

Showtime: The main radiation wing is underground...the waiting room. My fellow cancerees. I appear to be the youngest patient, and again I notice that there are no children at all. An elderly woman is wheeled past in hospital bed, withered, unable to rise. Children playing with toys, apparently waiting for father. We're all in it together.

A tech calls my name and I go to a secondary waiting room, change my shirt for a gown. Then into the radiation room itself. Funny, it looks just like the simulation room. What if they made a mistake: what if they radiated me the first time and this is the simulation?

Two techs help me down onto the table. There's a sheet on it and they tug on it, one side then the other, while my eyes widen. That's how bad it is: I'm afraid of a bed sheet moving under me. The radiation head, or whatever it is, of the linear accelerator is right over my face: the staff has taped "inspirational" and "wacky" pictures to it: snaps of pets, children, aphorisms: *One foot in front of the other. A smile is God's way of washing your face.*

They turn the lights out and for a moment there's a display grid running across my bare chest: numbers and lines. It's like laser tag, or a laser sight, they're lining me up in the crosshairs, for what will be two separate doses of relatively brief duration. I know it's time for the real deal when the techs get the hell out of the room.

No, Mr. Bond, I expect you to die.

Okay, this is it. Los Alamos time. The head of the accelerator swivels around me, and there's a general buzzing noise from the equipment. I don't feel a thing, or see anything either. The head swivels back around me and the first session is done. The techs come back for round two.

Well, that didn't take long. Maybe this radiation stuff isn't so bad. Except when the techs help me up off the table. Zotz! I feel such a twist in the small of my back, that knife in my vertebrae given a twist. But I appear to be alive and non-glowing.

It's only after I have my shirt back on, and I'm walking back to the main reception area, that I feel it. Ow...something's going on down there. My mom and sister are out there with a wheelchair, like they've read my mind (or my spine) and I really need to sit down in it. Every minute hurts more. My mom wheels me out and I need to wait. Man do I feel it now: crumpled, like a football team cleated over my spine. Today I am a cancer patient. I sit there, head in hands, waiting for this to pass.

Margot says, "Take another painkiller."

Sure, and another and another. I am so sick of this.

Home.

***

NEXT DAY: SECOND DOSE OF radiation.

How can I describe radiation therapy? The linear accelerator, what is the name of it? Like a giant mixmaster, uh, without the bowl and with the blades. Or like an electric can opener, without the blades. Sort of. The pictures taped underneath, of employees, dogs, children, inspirational stickers.

There is a waiting area outside the treatment room. I am directed to a second area that is obviously the workplace of more religious employees, indicated by the religious signage. Both in the waiting room and on the accelerator. It's annoying to me and I wonder if a patient ever protested.

Lunch. Then, marrow biopsy. A nurse preps me, showing me pictures of needles and devices, explaining the procedure in detail. "Most people say that the only thing they really feel is the suction, that that's the only pain. You'll feel it all down the leg. Some people say that it's really weird, like nothing they've ever felt before, like their leg is being emptied out from inside."

Okay, okay, I get the picture. Is she for real?

Ativan tablet under the tongue. Anesthetic. Some sort of IV drip. Here comes Doctor S.

"I have a hair-trigger spine," I explain nervously. For this is what I'm most worried about—that my bones will snap in the stress of the procedure.

I'm presented with a three-ring binder, a CD selection (not an iPod or mp3s, but actual CDs someone will load into a player), and it's not bad...I pick Beethoven's 7th, always good in a pinch.

Well, I can't look. I feel the pinch of the anesthetic injection, the eventual spread of the numbing puddle. The doctor is fiddling. "How does that feel?"

"How does what feel?"

The doctor laughs. "That's the right answer."

I can't look. Presumably a harpoon is now wedged into my pelvis. The Ativan is dissolving under my tongue, slightly chalky. Ludwig V... impressions...I'm so miserable, close to tears, but I will not cry. The nurse has my shoulders in her hands and is massaging them, I would rather she didn't but I'm in my little cocoon, my little escape pod, and I don't want to come out. I'm dropping down a well, into a world where a doctor is not sucking out my bone marrow with a needle.

Except that he is. The big moment has arrived and the doctor is speaking to me, in a loud direct voice that cuts through the music and right to my mind. "All right, I'm going to take the sample now."

That nurse was right. It's like nothing I've ever felt before: an eerie live numbness running down my leg. And, unfortunately, it's like nothing I've ever heard before either. Through the Ativan, through the numbness, through the headphones and their piping music, comes the unmistakeable sound of a straw sucking a marrow shake: shhhhhlorp... and again shhhhlorp and again.

There's something else too: me saying *Ow*.

If you ever want to learn what a wine bottle feels like when it's being uncorked, this is how to do it.

They give me Zometa the next day, the bisphosphonate bone-strengthening drug. I spend nights at at my parents' staying on the sofa. The pillow. In a moment the sick room is assembled: the sofa, the pillow, the night table.

Zometa day: I hate this stuff. I'm only here cause I have to be, cause I have to get my cancer treated. What do you think, I come here for my health? It has to be given intravenously.

Thursday: another day of radiation.

Chapter Eight

PROGENY

THIS IS ONE OF THE unlikelier aspects of myeloma, I suppose. Since it tends to be diagnosed in people of middle-age or older, the aspect of its treatment (via thalidomide) having to affect children or the possibility of having children is not one that is majorly discussed. And even people at my age have often finished having any children they may want.

After one or two false leads involving some awkward (for me) phone calls to various clinics and hospitals in the Delaware Valley, I finally locate Sperm Central, a reproductive center in downtown Philadelphia. This is what I'm looking for: the place to bank my pre-thalidomized sperm on ice in the event I find someone delirious enough to bear my children.

A date and time for my first appointment are set, the fees are laid out: $500 for the initial visit/interview/sample donation, then a reduced fee for any follow-up visit needed if the initial sample isn't up to scratch, and an annual fee for every year my deposits remain with the clinic. (I believe the frozen assets joke has already been played). Naturally my insurance won't cover any of this; I'll be paying for the sperm bank out of pocket, so to speak.

One crucial point of my first contact with the clinic remains, made by the efficiently cheerful woman on the phone: "You have the option of donating your sample in our offices, or you can do it at home and bring it in."

This may not be news to some of you readers, but I'm good and stumped by this for a moment. Bring it in? "At what point after I've generated my sample should I bring it in?"

"As quickly as possible. Right away, as a matter of fact."

I should like to point out that we are in the middle of winter. I'm supposed to transport my sample through the freezing streets of Philadelphia? At what point does the "good freezing" of the sperm bank become the "bad freezing" of the open air? I presume I couldn't masturbate into an ice cube tray in my kitchen, then stroll leisurely over to the clinic, tray in hand, as if on my way to a potluck dinner. Even if it was summer out, isn't the stuff going to dry or otherwise "go bad" before the clinic does whatever clinical stuff it needs to do? Like most men (I presume) once I've taken care of business, I want to spend as little time as possible dealing with the aftermath. I don't really want to have to engage in a juggling act/race against the clock.

Let's just say I want this wank-session to be as clinical as possible. I establish that there is a room set aside for sample collections, and make a date.

Which just happens to be January 15th, the Rev. Dr. Martin Luther King's birthday holiday. The clinic is open for business that day; fertility, or the pursuit of same, waits for no one. But my office/school is closed, so—no disrespect to Dr. King—I've taken advantage of that fact to slot a series of appointments into that day. Besides the fertility clinic, I'll be picking up a back brace at a medical supply store in town (DAS BACK...what's German for back or spine?), then heading to Northeast Philadelphia for an afternoon appointment at Fox Chase, to have blood drawn for HLA-marrow testing. This will test compatibility of my immune system with with my sisters' to see if one of them could be a bone marrow donor for my transplant. Quite a day, and I've arranged to be at the fertility clinic first thing in the AM to make sure I can fit everything in.

So to speak.

All during these arrangements there has been one especially bothersome fact troubling me, namely performance anxiety. You know you really have problems when you are worried about whether or not you can masturbate. But worry I do: as previously noted, regular 20 mg doses of OxyContin have been having their side effects. Little to no sexual desire at all, no morning wood, nothing. I have not had an honest-to-goodness erection in weeks.

I've resolved to skip the dose of OxyContin that morning but 1) what guarantee do I have that this will do any good? Doesn't that stuff linger in your system for a while? Should I skip the previous evening's dose too? 2) Assuming I skip the dose and my libido gets a chance to rebound, what about my back? Will that start hurting so much that I won't be able to concentrate? Fire away? How many doses should I skip? What if I can't sleep the night before? How humiliating would that be, to have to walk out of the donor room empty-cupped?

Even though I've described my general health situation to the one clinician by phone, I didn't go into the details of my pain- (and plea-sure-)killer problem. And what kind of ejaculation will I have anyway? Will I wash away the clinic with a month's backed-up tidal wave of jizz, or will anything come out at all? Is it all used up?

***

*D*AY DAWNS, AS IT OFTEN does. I had taken my OxyContin the night before, so I manfully forego it that morning. Now I've heard the stories about sperm banks, how they've got porn mags and sometimes even porn flicks to help out donors, but I'm not taking chances. I print out a particularly effective porn story I've found and saved online and tuck it in my bag.

Cold out. Take a cab. I don't want to be late for my date. You only get one chance to make a good first impression! Also it's too cold out and my back (are you ready for this?) is killing me.

When I enter the clinic, I realize I am the only single male there. The reception area is filled with women. Well, of course, anyone but an idiot would have realized that ahead of time. The only men beside myself are there with women, their spouses, their significant others. Nobody looks anybody in the eye: there seems more discomfort, less camaraderie than I have ever experienced in a doctor's office. There's a sense that we're all losers, that if we were functional and normal we wouldn't have to be here.

So my name is called, I get to the main desk and fill out my forms, answer the questions.

"Did you bring your sample with you?"

Groan. I thought we'd resolved all this ahead of time over the phone. No, I say. I didn't. I figured I'd....

Out comes the cup and a peel-off label, which the woman at the counter sticks on the cup. She doesn't seem too happy, as if I'm fouling up her day or something.

"Follow me, please."

She leads me down the hall and there it is, the sample room, inspirer of a million dirty jokes and speculations. The sperm donor room. I feel as if I'm being introduced to a farmer's daughter. What, you really exist? I thought people just made this up for laughs.

"Please write your name and date on the label. And when you're finished, bring the sample back to us."

The small plastic cup, about the size of an individual serving of pudding. Well, at least it's got a wide mouth. I was worried I was going to have to target a test tube and make a mess of things.

So here I am, in the place of legend, the sperm donor/masturbation room. It's about the size of the dorm rooms I remember from college— and, really, what's the difference?

There's an easy chair, a small low table with magazines, a TV/DVD unit chained to the wall, a sink, a toilet. Can you feel the love? I examine the magazines, and to my chagrin find nothing but FHM? *FHM?* Who do they expect to be using this room, nothing but 14-year-olds? This is not going to do it. The misery of imagining that I won't be able to produce. That I won't even be able to masturbate. There is a tape loop of despair running just under things.

Let's see what's on TV...I switch on the set and the DVD, get the disc going. What do you know, the TV is on permanent mute. I punch the volume button on the remote, but there's nothing. The sound on the set has been switched permanently off. How am I supposed to follow the plot of the movie now?

Sure, okay, I understand. The staff doesn't need the embarrassment of a porn soundtrack blasting through the closed door of the donation and out into the hall. We all know what's going on in there, no need to rub it in while some guy's rubbing one out, I can see the reasoning behind that...But, come on, there is this invention called headphones, would it bust the clinic's budget to throw a set of headphones in here?

I am paying $500.00 for this appointment. For $500 I could get really good and laid with a decent escort, never mind buying a set of head-phones. How am I supposed to follow the plot? By reading lips? Which ones?

And now I discover that the fast-forward function on the DVD player isn't working either, which is a problem, because the DVD is off to a really slow start. We haven't even got past the phone-sex ads yet. Phone sex ads with no sound, what a turn-on. I'm jabbing that fast-forward button like I mean it. Silent phone-sex ads! All right, forget it. I switch off the set in disgust. What else can you expect from an or-ganization run by caring, competent, sensitive, professional women? A lousy selection of pornography, that's what! No sense of pornography at all. I see I'm on my own here in the masturbation room. I have to do everything myself.

There is only one thing in my favor, and that is the fact that I have not had an orgasm in weeks. Somewhere behind my cancer, behind the pain and the medication for the pain, there is life, the force that drives the green fuse, etc.

I still have my printed-out story in my bag. Somehow I had a feeling it would be useful. I can't say why I didn't bring a magazine, a real porn magazine...I suppose I didn't want to cart it around with me all day. And (take note) it's always easier to hide thoughts in words than in pictures.

I've read the story before, of course, more than once. I know how it goes, but something about it appeals to the keystone of me, the reptile brain (you know it when you feel it) and I busy myself, after first won-dering exactly where I'm meant to stand, finally I take a stance by the sink, seems the logical place...and I busy myself, and the story begins to work, it's so filthy, and I begin to feel something, it's like the first moments of waking as the real world and its light begin to penetrate through your sleep. And you know you're back someplace well-known.

There is not a lot of sensation. My back hurts. I am still fuzzed by OxyContin: it feels like there is a net of webbing just under my skin, obscuring everything. But my life has been held back so long now, there is no holding it back any further. What happens next has little or nothing to do with pleasure, but with plain physics, raw anatomy. I am not halfway to an erection before I ejaculate, a painful miserable wonderful release. My jangled head. I am, mostly, relieved I was able to do this. Smearing myself into the cup. Is this enough?

The idiotic DVD has been running silently behind me. I switch it off, then carefully screw the lid on the cup and make myself presentable. I can't look the woman in the eye when I hand over the sample. The clinic is not done with me yet, though. To my surprise, I have to go into another room, get blood drawn, answer medical questions. Why wasn't this done first? Did they think it would really put me out of the mood? I'm exhausted now, these people have really drawn it out of me: sperm, blood. And the thing is, you don't even know the result. Before I leave, I make sure to swallow my reward, my 20 mg of painkiller. I see the miserable smear of myself in the cup...how could a child possibly arise from that?

I hope my popsicle kid appreciates everything I'm doing for him or her.

Later that day I'm at Fox Chase having more blood drawn, left arm this time, for marrow-donor testing. That's two blood-draws and a sperm-shot all in one day, MLK Day 2006. I have a dream.

A few days later, I get the call at work: the clinic was able to get 5 discrete vials from my overall sample. The ideal is ten, so it's strongly suggested that I visit again, repeat my experience. Sperm, let it slide.

So I'll be going back to do this all again, and under that as well, the ding-dong mantra in my skull: I have waited too long, I have waited too long. You're 44 years old, and your only serious attempt at fatherhood is whacking off into a plastic cup. Why don't I just cut my fucking throat?

Self-loathing: no one does it better than me.

Chapter Nine

BACKBONE

*I*T'S ALL ABOUT CONNECTIONS. NOT just the backbone connected to the hipbone and so forth, but who you're related to and married to and to whom who you're married to is related and so on. In this instance, besides my older sister Margot, who's a nurse practitioner (NP) at a leading cancer center, I've got the younger sister Judith, who's married to the head of orthopedic research at a prominent local university hospital. And who set up an appointment with a leading orthopedic surgeon. A back man.

SLEEPING: For a long time I do not go to bed at all. Since my two major pain experiences occurred getting out of bed, I was terrified to return there. Mentally I simply refused. So I slept on the sofa for weeks. Turned out I wasn't doing my back any favors: not straight and so on. Being bent: no good. So I was aggravating my back and prolonging the pain.

Finally, on the night of January 13, I couldn't take it anymore. I got up in the middle of night and got into bed, then fell asleep quickly and had the best sleep ever.

I always knew deep down that would happen, seeing the way the way I'd almost fallen asleep on pad during radiation. Then in the morning, I have a full bladder and am afraid to get up, feeling the twinges. I actually consider pissing myself, or as an alternative dumping my water glass out on the floor (as easier to clean up) and pissing in the glass.

Finally I start the process of wriggling out. Pain, yelling out, but not the worst. I really feel that bladder as I maneuver onto my stomach. Out and out, to squatting position, up on my feet. Okay, I've got a system. I finally realize I should put that piss bottle to use.

Saturday night, January 14: Success with bed. I am able to get out of bed with no twinges at all. Best morning ever! Don't even take the morning painkiller!

So it appears that if I can keep from aggravating the back, I'm way ahead of things. It was the constant aggravation of my back that was annoying me, caused by the sofa. But if I lie flat, no problem. And using the piss jug is a brilliant idea: no need to get out of bed and wake up fully, just drain. This Sunday morning is the best morning since this whole shit-trek began. The best is not having to take the OxyContin. My cock responds! I'm human! I'm back!

THE BACK: At its worst, what does it feel like? The grinding of the bones. I feel like I'm all exposed skeleton from shoulders to pelvis, like Itchy, the hard-luck cat on *The Simpsons*, after Scratchy has pulled another ghoulish trick on him. No skin, no muscle, no organs, just exposed spine and ribs with my living head grimacing on top, and those bones grind and grind in the naked air. You could throw a rock at me and ding my vertebrae. Step right up. I'm open. That grinding.

What does it feel like when I'm trying to get out of bed? Horrible. Like my pelvis is a cinder block and my spine is a single strand of limp spaghetti trying to hold it up, a single limp strand of spaghetti scotch-taped to the top of a fifty-pound cinder block and it's not going to hold for long. That's my spine.

Chapter Ten

THE SISTERS SPEAK

MARGOT: By way of introduction, I am the older sister, who works as an NP. There were so many times during ER visits, hospitalizations, emergency surgery and "near death" events when I almost wished I didn't have the medical knowledge to know how bad things were for my brother.

The next few chapters give Joshua's point of view during the various stages of treatment, but he was often so sick from the disease itself and the side effects of the drugs that he lost big chunks of time. I'll give a brief explanation here of what the treatment stages were to clarify what was happening.

RADIATION

The radiation therapy that Joshua received was aimed at reducing his bone pain by eliminating the plasmacytomas in his vertebrae. This would not affect the overall course of the disease, since the malignant cells would still be produced in his bone marrow, but it would help alleviate the worst symptom of pain.

INDUCTION

Joshua's initial treatment was started to get his M-spike number into the normal range by reducing the number of monoclonal, malignant plasma cells. The doctors told Joshua that he would not be getting "chemotherapy," meaning that he would not be receiving drugs that had to be delivered intravenously through slow infusion. The drugs he took to reduce his plasma cell numbers were all taken orally; nonetheless, their side effects were serious.

There are a variety of drug combinations that can be used to kill the wayward plasma cells of myeloma. One of the most effective treatments is a combination of thalidomide and dexamethasone. Thalidomide is the drug that became infamous in the 1960s for causing limb-shortening birth defects in babies whose mothers took it during pregnancy. The same properties that make it bad for a fetus make it effective against cancer: it is anti-angiogenic and anti-proliferative (inhibits blood vessel growth and cell division). It works in synergy with the powerful corticosteroid, dexamethasone, to cause a significant response in the majority of multiple myeloma patients.

Both drugs have serious side effects. Besides its potential as a teratogen, thalidomide can cause deep vein thrombosis (DVT) and periperhal neuropathy (hands and feet going numb), as well as severe fatigue and constipation. Dexamethasone causes mood disturbances in almost everyone and actual psychosis in some. Many people on Dex feel hyper and energetic, but often anxious with a hair-trigger temper as well. As the drug wears off, there is a "crash" with severe fatigue and depression, and sometimes suicidal thoughts. Dex suppresses the immune response to infections and patients can get new infections as well as reactivations of old, dormant infections; diseases such as chickenpox are life-threatening to someone on Dex.

*T*RANSPLANT

The thalidomide/Dex treatment isn't a cure, or even a chance for a total remission. The only hope for total remission in myeloma is a stem cell transplant (SCT), also called a bone marrow transplant. SCTs can be autologous (coming from the patient) or allogeneic (coming from a donor).

Part of the transplant planning back then involved my sister and me having blood drawn and typed for human leukocyte antigen (HLA) to see if either one of us could be a stem cell donor for Joshua. As it happened, neither one of us matched him (though we matched each other), so he was prepared for an autlogous transplant.

For an autologous SCT, one's own stem cells are removed from peripheral blood before the transplant, by a process called apheresis. The cells are stored and then used after the induction is complete. In Joshua's case apheresis was done about 10 days before the planned SCT hospitalization. At transplant, the patient gets high-dose chemotherapy, a drug called Melphalan, to kill the myeloma cells. The stored stem cells are then infused back to the patient through the catheter after the Melphalan infusion.

Melphalan is a chemotherapeutic drug that attacks all fast-growing cells, not only cancer cells but also cells of the lung, gut, liver, kidneys, and mucosa—and, of course, the bone marrow. In the period between treatment and the engraftment of the transplant, the transplant recipient is susceptible to bleeding (lack of platelets) and, most importantly, to infection (lack of neutrophils, the infection-fighting white cells, a condition called neutropenia). The average period of neutropenia after autologous SCT is 12 days, and the length of this period correlates strongly with infection.

I kept my eye on those numbers throughout the process. An absolute neutrophil count (ANC) of 0 or a platelet (blood clotting) count of 6 would send me into quiet, internal hysterics and a feeling that my head would explode if Joshua's numbers didn't start rebounding soon.

Chapter Eleven

INDUCTION

THALIDOMIDE THE BOWLING BALL, MY THOUGHTS THE PINS

SATURDAY GOT A LITTLE NASTY towards late afternoon: Onset of stomach upset in the Tuscany café with a friend. The dark, the wet, the winter cold and wind don't help. Seriously bad, the wind frightens me. I hang out in Barnes & Noble, get a diarrhea attack. Then about an hour later, again on South Street, heading to a restaurant, South Street Souvlaki (which is closed), bad flip of the stomach, turning inside out, my coat too thin. Cancer, winter, cold, it's bad. Feeling the bad side. My thin coat, the wind, the dark, the crowds I cannot join. So grateful for the open bathroom. That guy who makes me shut the door, I know I've seen him before. He has a point but he seems like a prick.

Year of Magical Thinking.

Body World's exhibit, work in. That was January 14, Saturday.

I'll remember it to my dying day. Which shouldn't be too much of an effort, heh heh, my timeline being what it is.

Talk about Thalidomide. The process of ordering. The pharmacy.

My co-pay with my prescription plan is $15.00. I'm curious.

"Humor me," I ask the pharmacist. "What would this cost me without insurance?"

She looks at the attached slip. "Six thousand eight hundred and eighty dollars."

Ha ha, no really. What would it cost?

She shows me the slip. There's the figure right in front of my eyes: $6680.09. I cannot believe it. Of all the things I've heard in the past month, this is perhaps the most astonishing. Seven thousand dollars? For these pills? What do they expect you to do if you have no coverage? Pay for all this? How on earth is a person supposed to pay for all this? I start trying to add up the costs of my treatment so far, the visits, the radiation, the other meds, figures I never actually bothered to check. I have no idea but suppose I'm well into five figures. And I'm not even dead yet! I'll have to keep on paying! And what about the cremation costs? The will? Things I really will have to pay for? Goddamn, this shit is lethally expensive!

What about the fucking stem cell transplant? People could just drop dead! And, in my swaddled cocooned existence, this situation has never once occurred to me. What do you do if you have no health coverage? You're completely fucked!

***

*D*RUGS: DEXAMETHASONE. THALIDOMIDE. ZOMETA. OXYCONTIN/ OXYCODONE.

Dexy's midnight runner (Come on, I lean). The little green pills. Chalky. The burn, the burning fuzz. Stokehole in brain. Lighthouse brain, whirling bulb. The dull unblinking brain. (It's not like I'm really focusing on anything, I just can't shut the thing down). Can I hear my bones? The way I heard my mucus in my chest, shifting marshily? Why not listen all the way down, hear everything: marrow, bone, organs, my hair as it grows, my skin as it sheds. My bowels harder than Hoover Dam. The pin-prickles of yellow light as I blink my eyes: OxyContin. My sensitive teeth. My curling toes. Did I just feel my shin ripple?

Thalidomide: Serious med time. The NP reads me the riot act about Thalidomide. Here it is, item by item. Birth defects. Drowsiness. Nerve damage. Water retention. Bloating. I think I'll stick to the cancer, thanks. They're serious about this stuff. Registration number. I'll have to phone into a database. And so on and so forth.

The packets, the pills. The text: And just for all you illiterates out there, the Thalidomide people have added a helpful picture of a deformed (and smiling) baby, foreshortened limbs and all.

Here comes Cancerman, waddling down the sidewalk. Get a load of me: plastic bag in one hand, free hand out in a kind of airy paddle, balancing me as I make my way. I'm living my 60s in my 40s. The brace under my clothes pads me out. You think I care what I look like? I don't fucking care.

***

*D*EATH OF A LAPTOP: FIRST week of January

The blur, the hours, the days. The only thing I care about when I'm out is getting back home. The best comfort I've taken is on my sofa with a blanket wrapped around me. I resent my job. I resent my doctors. I resent my medicine. I resent having to make appointments, request insurance referrals, pick up prescriptions, get prescriptions filled, having to do physical therapy exercises. Every little thing I have snags on something else. Every article of clothing snags on something. I resent having to talk.

And the rage. Have to watch the rage, especially at work. Borderline psychotic, reliving old feuds, twenty years distant and more...the resentment, the crankiness. I really have to watch that. As soon as I'm at work, all I can think about is getting through the hours until it's time to go home. I figure I hauled my tired ass out of bed and got it into the office in a reasonable time, now you expect me to *work*, too? Fuck that! You assholes are lucky I'm even here. But the job sustains my medical coverage.

I'm getting used to the Thalidomide. It's a happy day when Dr. S tells me I can stay at 150 mg dosage, on account of good blood results. Because I am finally used to it.

NEWS EVENTS: The miners, dead then alive then dead. Brokeback Mountain. Iraq. Bush...President Bush is on TV, lying his ass off. The sound is down, but I can see his lips moving, so there's no doubt about it. Cheney shoots Whittington. More Iraq.

How much better Nick Cave sounds when you have cancer!

Am I hooked on OxyContin? How would I know? I'm afraid to ask the doctors. The ache, the sweats, the feverish feeling.

First time at the multiple myeloma support group. The blizzard. Falling asleep later that night.

Hamster wheel: realizing that whatever aggravation I can attribute to "bad luck," still it only brought out what was already in my personality,

like cancer cells waiting to be triggered. Surliness, emotional cruelty...
now I was "justified."

My laziness. The story of the orangutan that sits dreamily for hours,
then solves the intelligence test at once, puts the right peg in the right
hole.

To be a drop, to enter the stream.

Bromides. People want to hear of angels....only a human would
invent an angel. Why would an angel look like a human?

***

WHICH WAY I FLY IS HELL, MY SELF AM HELL

The greatest achievement in the entire trace of English literature,
in the course of the language itself, four words, four syllables!, arrayed
just so to convey the maximum weight of universal anguish. My. Self.
Am. Hell. Brilliant! There's no place else to go, folks! You can't escape
yourself, we've all tried, but all attempts to do so only make your self
worse, there is only one thing to do and those who've accomplished it
aren't talking. My head on fire, my skull burning, Nick Cave's mercy
seat, and I fear my head is burning, and I feel my blood is raining...

Yes, I see it now, a whole new genre of fiction to create and exploit,
a fresh new market, novel for the blood-cancer crowd. Plate-lit:

BRIDGET JOSH'S DIARY

Monday 6 March

142 lbs. (v.g., losing ever more weight by the day, yay cancer!), Dexamethasone units 10, Thalidomide units 3 (all as prescribed, am being
v.g. outpatient, if more than a little groggy), OxyContin units 2 (20 mg
every 12 hours: remember to swallow and not chew), cigarettes 0 (fat
sodding load of good that's done me), alcohol units 0 (who needs booze
when you've got OxyContin and thalidomide?!), IgG level...x, M-spike: x

There's a faint glimmer of an erection this morning as I awake on
the sofa. I don't bother with it and slink off with my tail between my
legs (so to speak), as is the usual state of affairs these days. I drink the
water I'd remembered to leave within arm's reach on the window sill,
pop my morning Oxy, and away I go—pushing off the sofa, huffing
with backache, shuffling to the toilet to see if my blockaded bowels will

move. Of course they do not. I'll likely hear from them while on the subway to the office.

No e-mail from Ann this morning. She doesn't love me anymore. Must remember to phone her today/tonight, must remember not to grumble/shout in my usual dex-inspired frustration, as I did last time (might this have something to do with no e-mail from her?).

I paddle-walk up to 2nd and Market for the subway. Make it into the office only 20 minutes late: excellent. My bowels are finally motivated to speak out after a second cup of coffee; I marvel at the elongated result before flushing.

The day passes in the usual fuzz: making website updates, attempting to "focus" on "long-time projects." Hello, don't you people know I'm on cancer medication? Oh, that's right, I'm still keeping this a secret from everyone but my immediate superior and the office manager.

I curse when I have to set up the laptop-projection system in the conference room, which requires physical exertion on my part. I return e-mails with as little commitment as possible to actually promise to do what the e-mailer requested. At noon, I shuffle to the corner grocer/convenience store for a great take-out soup to supplement lunch.

Still no e-mail from Ann.

I'm home in time for the 6 PM OxyContin, just ahead of the squeezy/achy feeling inside and in my ribs. I can feel it kicking in as dinner begins to defrost. Oh yeah.

8 PM: the magic hour, when 20 mg of time-released OxyContin has fully kicked in, and last night's bedtime dose of Thalidomide (150 mg) has mostly filtered out of my system in advance of tonight's dose. Phew. I'll just sit on the sofa, catch up on a little reading before phoning Ann and turning out the lights.

11 PM: Uh oh. I wake up after my third "inadvertent nap" of the week. The lamp is burning in my face. I pop Thalidomide caps and phone Ann, leaving a lame apologetic message on her voicemail. Then I fumble off my clothes, fling them to the floor, draw up the ever-present blanket, arrange all the pill bottles that might possibly be needed within arm's reach if I'm dying in the middle of the night, switch off lamp, hit the sofa, fade.

Ta. Kew. Fanks very much.

Robert Lowell, New Year's Day:

"Again, and then again...the year is born/to ice and death." Poor Bob. He didn't get to stick around long enough for global warming. My bones are crackers. Dip my skeleton in your soup and watch it dissolve.

Chapter Twelve

APHERESIS ME TO PIECES

*I*REMEMBER MUCH LESS THAN HALF of what happened, or feel like
I've forgotten so much (but maybe I haven't?) and the parts I
do remember, I want to forget, so let's just forget it, okay?

Let's do it this way and imagine bringing in sand, umbrella, beach
chair to the hospital...resort.

To get to the stem cell transplant, the SCT, my stem cells were
needed. My own stem cells would be removed from my blood before
the transplant via the apheresis process, stored, and then used at the appropriate time. All the action takes place through a big catheter, placed
into a large vein in my chest, near the clavicle, in a radiology procedure
room with sedation. In my case, apheresis was planned about ten days
before SCT hospitalization. My harvested cells would be stored until
they were needed for the transplant, then infused back to me after I'd
been given high-dose chemotherapy to kill the myeloma cells.

Thursday, June 8. OK, this is really it, the ball has dropped, Elvis
has left the building and the show is getting on the road. They need a
chest x-ray before the catheter placement (for a baseline to make sure
they don't puncture a lung in the process) and right off the bat there's
a problem with referral.

They send me down to the x-ray/radiology department and the lady at the front desk gives me a hard time about my not having a referral, and it seems I can't win, here we go again—first step of the process and already there are insurance problems.

I get shown a phone and try to get through the voicemail system to my GP's office, and when they answer, they tell me my hospital is out of the network and blah blah blah. So here I am fucked, can't even get out of the dugout, can't even get my first procedural x-ray here without running into problems.

I'm freaking out, trying to plead my case, and they won't give me the referral, there's just no dice. I go back to the lady at the desk and tell her this, and she says if that's so then looks like no x-ray for me.

That's when the guy at the next desk/window politely butts in and asks to see my records. He declares that I've already been cleared for take-off by the insurance company: the x-ray is part of the transplant procedure which in its entirety has been cleared by the insurance company. No referral needed, I can pass GO without coughing up $200. The woman apologizes, and I'm not angry with her, not when I see how genuinely embarrassed she is by all this. It's okay; God knows how many mistakes and miscalculations I've made at my own job.

I wouldn't even be boring you with this whole fucking little interlude, except that when I go into the x-ray room to get the chest x-ray that I can't even remember what the fuck it was so necessary for, the technician—a sad-faced, careworn, paunchy fellow much shorter than my hunched-over self—makes small talk with me about my condition. In the course of things he mentions that his wife has just been diagnosed with ovarian cancer, and I can't think of a thing to say except to tell him how sorry I am and that I hope his job (is this the lamest thing to say or what?) allows for his wife to receive the best available care at the least expense.

I can't remember what he says to that; only how sad and methodical he was, and as I'm leaving he says, "Beat this thing!" and that's what I remember.

There's also the EKG, then Dr. S and his nurses laying out the apheresis schedule for the next few days, and the timing before I come into the hospital for the transplant. This is it, the SS *Poseidon* has set sail.

The next day, I go to Penn Tower for my first shot of Neupogen—a white blood cell "growth" factor to get my bone marrow revved up. The first shot is administered by nurse, but then I get the the weekend's worth of doses in a cooler, pre-loaded syringes to be kept in the fridge. I'm also told how medical supplies are due to be delivered for the home nurse who will tend to my catheter.

I start to feel a little weird on the way home, a little lightheaded. My stomach feels off; not nauseated, but like I don't want anything down there if I can help it. Poor appetite. Plus the fringes of panic. Like a rocket launch, we've entered the final countdown and this is really it, no backing out now, not without totally humiliating myself and inconveniencing a bunch of hardworking people.

Speaking of which, that afternoon I caught a screening of *An Inconvenient Truth*, the Al Gore global warming documentary, which I confess I went to more because I wanted to squeeze a movie in before my hospital adventure began than because I wanted to see it. I have to admit it's difficult for me to care; I've been convinced for some time that global warming is a fact, and that even if human activity is not directly responsible for it, we ought to err on the side of caution in that regard and proceed accordingly. I can sure pick the cheery movies to see just before a hospital stay....

***

CATHETER DAY

Up at 5:30...the day creeps up. Time seems tight even without eating breakfast. Down to the apheresis unit, where I'm supposed to be at 7:30, but find out they don't open till 8. I'm tired from no food or coffee and from the OxyC. Finally they draw blood, more than half a dozen vials.

You fuckers, haven't you drained enough blood from me by now? The idiot tech fucks up my right arm so they move to my left. With the crazy red gauze bandages, I look like something from the French Revolution.

Then it's time for the catheter to be implanted. It had been explained to me that something like a big cannula or intravenous line would be placed into a large vein in my upper chest and tunneled to stick out through my skin. It would be used during the apheresis and also during the transplant for infusions.

Despite the explanations, I was becoming more and more frightened as the moment arrived. This was my worst phobia: people are going to render me unconscious and then cut into me. What could be worse?

They are going to put something into me. It is going to stay there. All those surgical horror stories I used to hear about sponges, scissors, hangnails left in people after operations, and now I'm going to have an operation in which this is the point—not to take something bad out of me but to leave something artificial in? Help, a huge mistake is being made!

Off to registration and Radiology, where I really get nervous. I notice that my new patient file refers to lymphoma, not myeloma. They prep me for the catheter and I'm dismally nervous. I can't stand this stuff. I know what you people want to do, you want to make me unconscious and snip me up, why do you think they call it invasive procedure...

But it's not so bad, the doctors and nurses are pros, they're making small talk (sports, World Cup) and I feel as though I'm being rude. They know their stuff.

They're putting me under.

The last thing I remember is the vaguely sex-toyish battery-operated razor coming out to shave the chest hairs on my right side. Oh and the surgical resident with not only the surgical paper mask on but the plastic visor on, like a clear light plastic welder's visor. What, are you people expecting things to splatter? But before I can give that much thought, I'm out for the duration.

They wake me up, woozy; maybe you know how it is. I can't believe it's over. Dopey, anesthetized. There's a big bandage over my right chest that I don't pay much attention to, with a couple twinned inches of tubing poking out underneath, each with a plastic port on the end, one red, one blue. I'm so dopey this doesn't bother me much at the time. Folks meet me, then pick up Neupogen and an experimental drug AMD-3100 that may or may not help stimulate my bone marrow to "mobilize" more stem cells for the transplant. Be sure not to mix them up.

I ride out to my younger sister Judith's with her husband Lou, but have to make it back home in time for the nurse. Very uncomfortable. My mood grows worse at Judith's house. Judith's friend Abby, whose divorced husband died a while back, and her depressed kids all sadden me as I think of their griefs. I apologize for being such a downer. Lou gives me a ride back.

The visiting nurse arrives with the mystery drug, of which I am terrified. *Batman Begins* is on TV. The injection: it feels the same as Neupogen. The nurse is very nice and "talks me down," telling me not to worry too much about the drug, it's an approved drug—it just hasn't been used for marrow/apheresis before.

Apheresis takes place on Tuesday and Wednesday. The nurse was called off for Wednesday shots. Just chilling in the hospital Thursday, check out Friday. My queasy stomach, inability to sleep. I go over the second schedule, the real one, that I've been given, involving the transplant itself.

I can't remember Thursday. Did I leave the hospital on Thursday? I think I left on Friday, folks taking me home. We stop at Famous Deli for too much deli food. It's too heavy, but I'm so hungry I order a towering corned beef sandwich with potato salad. Too greasy; I can only eat half, and take the rest home, where the thing turns into a glistening flesh-sculpture with gelid spangles of fat in my fridge.

But I am obsessed with finishing it, consumed with eating it (ha ha). Which I do, to my gastric distress—but you know, I even come to enjoy that a bit, the knowledge that my system is active again, full, working, resistant. Always resistant.

What did I do that night? Who knows and it doesn't matter. E-mails, phone calls, DVDs, browsing newspapers. My concentration is totally shot, can't read a book.

The view from the window. The shot child, the news report. Zarqawi dead, Bush in Iraq. My myeloma has a better chance of being cured than Iraq has of finding peace and stability.

Packages start arriving from Amazon. A collegue at work had asked about my Wish List, alerting folks to it, so now there's a regular arrival of packages with their cards. Music CDs, Beethoven and Brahms, Etruscan marble-like box sets of DVDs: *Monty Python, Mr. Show, The Simpsons,* a variety of documentaries of musical acts. Oh and books, too. How to speak Arabic, military history....

Well, I'm all set, I think. There will never be a dull moment in the hospital or recuperating in my sister's house, I'm going to get so much done. Ha ha ha ha ha....

June 16 (Friday). The heat, the heat, already the heat. Yeah, surrrre global warming is a liberal conspiracy. The heat of that summer settling in, pressing in, the storms. I sit in all day reading, considering taking in the Bloomsday festivities across town, but simply too weak to make it. Probably spent a fair amount of time writing. Ha ha, wouldn't that be funny, to have it turn out that so much of the "lost time" I'm trying to regain was spent working on the first draft of this memoir. Ha ha, that would be hysterical. Napping, recuperating. Watching *Simpsons* DVDs probably. The sets of the second and third seasons will thrill my nephews.

June 17 (Saturday): Reading *The Plot Against America*. Began it the previous Saturday afternoon the 10th—or was it Sunday the 9th? I think it was Sunday, because that night the folks picked me up and we went to Penn, checked in, had dinner at New Deck Tavern. Saturday night was Tyler's photo-party, the Food and Beverage Party. People were smoking dope up in Tyler's attic. I can't remember if I smoked the dope myself. I don't think I did then, concerned enough about the painkillers I was still on and the alcohol.

June 18 (Sunday): I biked up to a gallery on 3rd Street to see a photo exhibit. The reason I went was that the exhibit included a couple of photos by a woman I had met at the party from the previous night. And there they were: interesting sepia-toned photos of Kenyan life, just like she said. Pieces of life fitting together in a pattern—a very sooth-ing notion just then. Not quite sure of the thought behind it: shots of modern Africans treated to look like the souvenirs of a hundred years before. To suggest that this is how the west will always view Africa? To recreate the past?

I'm the only person in the gallery. Have to cram my culture in before I disappear.

I seem to recall that I started watching *Youth of the Beast*, a Suzuki Yakuza film, on Saturday night. At some point I fell asleep, then watched the finish on Sunday, a routine fairly common during this period. Or maybe not, if I went to Ted's party that night. What differ-ence does it make?

Cut and run. Cunt and rue.

Okay, now I remember: at some point during all this, the Penn Health home care nurse comes to my place to show me how to tend to my catheter. A big box of supplies is delivered. Inventory: stubby syringes pre-loaded with saline flush; accessories pertaining thereto, including alcohol wipes, gauze, mask, plastic gloves. The multi-gallon red plastic disposal jug for the depleted syringes, complete with internal plastic collar to prevent used syringes from slipping back out. When I'm done with all this, I'm told, I am not—repeat NOT—to dispose of these materials in the routine trash. I am to call the health agency and someone will come to take it away, take the used syringes away like toxic waste, recycle the unused supplies.

There are also dressings for my catheter, for where it disappears into my chest, because that's got to be covered so it doesn't get infected. There is a constant low-grade alarm at all times now, like marshy ground underfoot, or a ringing in the ears. What I'm aware of is that my immune system is going to be deliberately destroyed very soon, so why was an easily infected plug placed into my chest?

The box, big enough for a TV, squats in my front room. An appointment is made for a catheter-cleansing tutorial: the nurse comes and patiently walks me through it, if that's the word, or injects me through it, or cleanses me through it. I'm a little embarrassed at first by the state of my apartment, but the nurse doesn't give it a glance, and I realize she's likely been all over the Delaware Valley and seen everything. I don't engage her in conversation, don't ask her about herself, because I just want this all to be over with as quickly as possible.

There is even a thick three-ring binder, with instructions and diagrams, thank goodness, because I'll never remember this stuff: how to flush the catheter, how to mask myself, how to dress my bandage and the implant area, how to keep from getting killed even apart from the transplant process.

I'm impressed most by the nurse, to whose counsel I listen without asking much. Is it fun to visit people's houses? Has it ever been dangerous? How many does she see in a day? What's the greatest contrast between homes she's seen in a day? In her entire career? Why is she so considerate of others, how did she get into such an occupation? She doesn't mind my dusty sofa, my unswept floor....

June 19 (Monday). Back out to Penn for my "secret" one-shot trip to the cancer psychiatrist, another Dr. S! I don't tell anyone I'm going. Why is "s" simply the supreme starting letter of so many sussurative words in the English language? Behold my CD collection: more bands start with "S" than any other letter.

Anyway...my session with Dr S. I had some notes I'd prepared beforehand, my outlined CV of depression and failure, but that's really not the issue here. I need to calm down. I want drugs.

Aside from a social worker guy Margot had me meet at Fox Chase, to whom I spoke with twice, I haven't been in any counseling in over ten years.

I can't sleep, I can't calm down. Naturally, as soon as she prescribes the drugs I want, I equivocate: Ambien, Clonazepem, Lexapro. Kennedy's been in the news for Ambien. As if I think there's some risk of me getting behind the wheel of a car while in the hospital for the transplant.

I feel myself on the brink, looking at that small woman behind a desk. How can she do it? THE NATURE OF THE THERAPIST: How can she face the emotional pain that comes through her door eight hours a day? She doesn't look too cheery. But what would I or any patient think if she was? We'd think she was insane. Empathy.

I don't remember what was said. She sat behind her desk, tiny, only head and shoulders visible, but always the focal point of the room. Small office, not a conference type room. I sit across, on the couch against the wall opposite the desk, sometimes getting up and pacing.

I can't say the psychiatrist's visit did any specific good, but it didn't hurt, and it helped a little to know that there was one more person within the medical/hospital system willing to listen to me whine.

And still the ceaseless thought: they're really going to do this to me.

Chapter Thirteen

THE TRANSPLANT

T
HE ENTIRE APHERESIS PROCESS INCLUDED my recent couple over-
nights in the hospital, but the main transplant event required
a scheduled hospital admission, a reservation to the specialized hematology oncology floor at Hospital of the University of Pennsylvania
(HUP).

I'd been hunkered in my apartment, first round draft pick style, A/C
cranked, suitcase locked and loaded, doing nothing but waiting for the
call from University of Pennsylvania hospital admissions department
signaling me to come in. What consumed me most was the thought
that somehow they might forget me, that my case would fall through
the paperwork cracks, that the call would never come, that I would
have to call them. That someone would answer my call and say *Joshua
Who?* That's just silly, of course: everyone knows that hospitals don't
make mistakes, especially concerning patient identity, especially not
on the day you're to be admitted for high-dose chemo and a blood-cell
transplant. But one can always hope....

Mid-afternoon, and the hospital was as good as its word, dammit.
The phone rang non-fictionally, and the pleasant-voiced woman on the
other end informed me that my room on Rhoads 7 was ready for my
arrival. I could check in any time.

Camp Marrow, here I come!

My bag was all packed, my bag had *been* all packed, and now there was nothing to do but relay the message to my folks, the only people in the universe available to drive me to the hospital on a Tuesday afternoon without a meter. They've been waiting around just like me—if we'd been more organized, we would have figured out a place to wait together, like, say, I dunno, my apartment for example. That would havve saved a bit of time, but you do the best you can when you're distracted, and so within the hour they come to pick me up.

There's my rolling travel case with my laptop and books and other life-support gizmos wedged inside, and my suitcase with too many clothes that my father insists on carrying downstairs, thump thump, one step at a time. He's got to do something and I let him, while my mother rags him out and asks him what the hell he thinks he's doing.

Outside the world is cooking nicely. The street gives noticeably under your shoes. There's a lot of attempted conversation as my mom drives us east—What did they tell you? What was the phone call like? that sort of thing.

We're midway across town, on the 1500 block of Lombard Street; my mom always has to take the slow route because that's what she knows. The folks are sitting up front, me in the back seat. For some reason the car is halted. Maybe traffic was beginning to thicken up on the street, warming up for rush hour. For whatever reason we're sitting there like a long, low duck when another duck thumps us from behind.

It's not a crash; the other guy couldn't have been doing much more than rolling forward absentmindedly. But it's a solid love tap nevertheless, a concussion I feel right in my lower back. I can't stifle the groan that comes.

Consternation, flusteration, general uproar. My mom gets the car over to the curb. The jolt in my back, the pain, has gone as quickly as it came. There doesn't seem to be anything newly broken, but all I can think is what a schmuck I am for putting all my bags in the trunk. That's where I've stashed all my painkillers and, for the first time in recollection, an emergency is at hand. So naturally for the first time the meds I've always kept on my person for such an emergency are right where I can't immediately get at them.

At this point, I'm expecting a big tub of hippo shit right outside the car door as I crawl out—but no, it's just the sun-softened pavement again.

Everybody stands around. The driver of the other is a male who doesn't look quite thirty. In fact, he looks mortified. It's a little too hot for a real argument, but his body language conveys culpability. There's no point in yelling.

I get the keys and go for the trunk like the drug addict I am, pawing out the stop-gap Oxys and throwing down a couple with a swallow of warm juice.

It's a little touching as I overhear my dad trying to make an issue out of this pointless accident, making a point of saying how we were on our way to the hospital, I'm about to have an operation, blah blah. The mug who hit us just keeps looking worse and worse. I feel sorry for him now; he didn't mean to do it, and I once did exactly the same thing to somebody else at a tollbooth over a decade ago, so maybe this evens things out.

Oh, I almost forgot the best part. We dialed 911 on my mother's cell like good citizens who want to report an accident they were a party to, and we waited close to half an hour and the police never showed up. Nothing, not even a patrol car passing by. And all four of us are white! Gotta love Philadelphia. Presumably the cops had their hands full totting up murder victims elsewhere in town.

So we exchange information and off we go to HUP.

Registration. Doesn't take too long, except they have the same mistake on file, citing my illness as lymphoma instead of myeloma. I have to go out of the patient registration area and across a corridor to the window where I pay my co-pay. Why, why aren't these things consolidated? Up to Rhoads, 7th floor. I introduce myself at the main desk.

I'm in a shared room in a corner where I go about getting settled. Putting things out, unpacking a little. I fish out my iPod and notice it's doing something I've never seen before. Some kind of maintenance check. Did the collision set this off, trigger it? Now I'm really aggravated, as I can't seem to make iPod stop. Really distracted. Like some idiot spoiled child I can't focus on anything else, as if this is the sum of the day's worst events. My iPod is broken! How can I go on?!

I would have a sensational view overlooking what would be the courtyard separating a number of hospital wings, if it weren't filled with what appear to be the buildings housing the power units running the same buildings. I'm looking straight down at the roofs of brick structures covered with vents and shafts duction units?

A nurse comes in and starts getting the lay of the land. We're discussing the accident, the possibility of an x-ray, but that's ruled out. I can't stop fiddling with the malfunctioning iPod, which pisses off the nurse.

Dad says of the car accident, "He screamed."

I insist I didn't scream. I groaned but I didn't *scream*.

I change into a hospital gown. My roommate, whom I scarcely recall at this point, is an older man. White hair, mustached, looks like the actor Sam Elliott. He is being treated for some form of cancer but I can't remember his name or what cancer he had. Already I've entered the taking notes mode. What the hell is the matter with me? He told me his name, he told me the sort of cancer for which he was being treated, and I can't remember a word he said, nor did I bother to write any of it down.

Dinner is chicken. "Wow, such an appetite," my mom says. This is the last time anyone will say that about me for a while.

Then they sneak up on me. While it's still daylight, nurses hustle in the World War I-style toxic agent Melphalan, hook me up to an IV, and let it drip. And that's when it all turns black....

***

I'M UP EARLY ENOUGH THE next morning. I can't believe the coffee they give me to drink for breakfast. Are you guys kidding? Nothing but brown water. I venture out of the room. I feel suspiciously unchanged. Nobody stops me. They've taken me off the IV so I take a circuit of the floor in my gown. I put a surgical mask on, because it makes me feel better. Like I'm taking the necessary precautions. At some point a nurse explains to me that I can roam as I wish, could go throughout the hospital if I wanted to, and I am now inclined to test this.

The next day I am moved to private room. I think this is a dodge to get around insurance issues, since I don't believe I'm really covered for a single room. I remember this fairly well, the first room being "swept" by nurses of belongings (is this where I lost my Ambien?) and me being led down the hall. In between puking episodes, I guess. I never see my ex-roommate again. Is he all right? Sorry I don't remember anything about you, buddy. Probably best for the both of us that we didn't have to share a toilet after that one night.

My next recollections are mingled, but all involve me vomiting. I do not have a single memory of vomiting into the toilet, probably because I never did vomit into the toilet. It was, after all, at least four steps from the bed, a good eight feet away. No, I'm always heaving into a basin as I lie in bed. Chronology disintegrates. Washed away on a tide of unease and medication. The staff (doctors and nurses) seem to be listening specifically to my complaints about stomach upset and diarrhea. They've heard it all before, just so much noise to them. There are bags on the IV; I do not know what they are. There are pills given me to swallow; I swallow them.

In fact, here's what I remember of THE TRANSPLANT ITSELF, the centerpiece of my hospital visit, the main event, as it were: I look up to see a blue plastic vat on a tray by the side of my bed. I'm lying down and can't see into the vat but I can see steam rising out of it. This must be what they use to defrost the cells. There are a couple of nurses or doctors or something and they take an immense plastic syringe out of the vat. In fact, it looks a lot less like a syringe and more like what a baker uses to squirt curly-cue frosting on top of a cake, an impression strengthened by the translucence of the syringe which allows me to see the strawberry-pinkish contents within. Hey, it's my stem cells! I haven't seen you guys since last week! How you doing? Good to see you again!

No really, the stuff looks like cake frosting, strawberry cake frosting in a baker's tub. For an insane moment I am certain the nurse holding the tube is going to squirt Happy Transplant to You across my sunken chest. But in fact I do not know what she did with the tube, or if there were other tubes, or how the transplant proceeded, because memory draws an absolute blank. They must have shot the stuff in through my catheter though it sure looked awful thick and sludgy to me, sure to clog up the catheter tubes. I must have fainted right away as soon as they got the nozzle near my skin.

How do you like that? The most important part of my entire hospital stay (I guess) and I remember about eight seconds of it.

Anti-nausea patch on neck. Scopalamine? It's all been obliterated.

Days of post-Melphalan. Some recuperation. Visitors: Parents, Mark, the chaplain, Margot and her boys, Judith. Lou starts making *New York Times* delivery. It couldn't have all been so bad, as I have records of e-mails sent, and recall walking around Rhoads floor. Reading (Mr.

Arkadin, *The New Yorker*) and watching some DVDs. Doing a little work on the laptop. So it wasn't all so bad.

Until July 3rd, when the infection set in.

A night of diarrhea. Dreams of it. A vision of a family in raincoats sloshing through a downpour of liquid feces, a family in nightwear/pajamas/raincoats in an endless downpour of feces, like the opening scene in *Singin in the Rain*. A dream, or a permutation of what was happening to me, soiling the bed through the night.

The lounge. With cable TV, VCR, DVD, Xbox. The people you see in the lounge. Everybody's horrible story. The couple I saw one night, asleep in each other's arms. My story is a drop in the ocean.

That's what I'm trying to tell you, good people: If I am going into elaborate and sickening and repulsive detail about my cancer, it is only to let you know how unsingular, how ununique it is. There are millions of stories like mine.

And that's only where cancer is concerned. Think of all the other sick people, horrible and morbid as it is. I am trying to stir your sympathy, folks, not for me but for the world's halt and infirm. I doubt I really have to do that though, if the point I'm making has any validity. Scratch anyone and they have a story to tell, if not of themselves than of a near one, a loved one, a friend. There was no shortage of patients on the 7th floor of Rhoads that I noticed.

Chapter Fourteen

THE SISTERS SPEAK II

MARGOT

Looking through the "retrospectoscope," I'm convinced that if Joshua's HLA typing had matched Judith's or mine and he HAD received our donor stem cells, he would have suffered the same serious complication but never would have survived. In the years since Joshua's diagnosis, studies have found that allogeneic transplants in multiple myeloma have higher initial mortality rates (up to 40%) than autologous transplants (just over 10%).

Even the autologous transplant was a hard road. Joshua's initial SCT started out routinely enough, but a few days into the hospitalization he began to complain that his belly was swelling, that he felt "pregnant" and it was starting to hurt. The situation deteriorated rapidly and hit rock bottom where it stayed for about 3 days. Joshua had a 50/50 chance of surviving the bowel infection, or typhlitis, that had developed. If his bowel ruptured or perforated then the chance of mortality would skyrocket. The surgical team had been consulted and was on standby. Joshua was taken down for x-rays and scans at regular intervals to assess for possible perforation. His belly ballooned and was taut with pain. The surgeons had an additional worry that there was incipient development of necrotic or dead bowel. All of this going on when his immune system had no defense.

Every time Joshua groaned, moaned or called out in pain I imagined he'd perforated. Assessment could be challenging with Joshua as he seemed to have a variant of dysesthesia—a heightened sensitivity of his skin. The guy who didn't complain a lot about all his bone fractures would scream when tape or a band-aid was pulled off of his skin. Combine that with having a nasogastric tube (NGT) in place to keep the stomach decompressed, and it made for a few miserable few days.

A lifetime ago my college roommate, also a nursing student, had emergency abdominal surgery and required an NGT. I will never forget her telling me that the surgical incision was nothing compared to the NGT—that the NGT was actually the worst part of the hospitalization.

After a few days Joshua's neutrophil counts slowly inched up, his abdominal distention gradually decreased, the NGT was removed and it was as though the black clouds passed and the sun was out again. Joshua continued to improve.

During his hospitalizations, one of the hardest aspects to deal with was Joshua's confusion, delirium and hallucinations, often accompanied by paranoia. These, to me, signaled that something was wrong, and I tried to get the medical and nursing staff to really understand that my brother would become a different person in the hospital—the inpatient Joshua. His uncharacteristic behaviors meant that something was off. Sometimes his kidney function was abnormal or his calcium level was high, affecting his mental state. Other times it was fever caused by neutropenia or the side effects of his medications. The following chapters give his point of view of events he struggled to remember.

Chapter Fifteen

THE INFECTION

URNS OUT THERE'S A REASON why hospital staff checks your temperature and blood pressure every two hours, even coming into your room in the middle of the night and waking you to do it: you might be sick. One week post-transplant and I wake in the middle of the night, soaked in sweat, confused, achy. My head falling and spinning. And without any recollection of having asked for help, I am surrounded by nurses and staff, I hear them explaining to me that I have a fever, and they are sandbagging me, tucking sandbags of ice into my armpits, draping one over my burning forehead. There's something wrong and they caught it.

I don't remember how it started. All I begin to recall is my belly bulging like a pregnancy, my hands clasped over it as I wail to the doctors bent over my bed, begging them to make the pain stop.

"Do you feel this?"

The doctors are probing the hill that my gut has become, and I don't know what's worse—the pain as their fingers probe my stomach, or the worried looks on their faces. They look more dubious than I feel, and I know something is seriously wrong.

"Do you feel this?"

Owwwwwwgh! Yeah I feel it! Uhhnnnnnnghh! Make it stop!

Here's what seemed to have happened. Some bug lurking in my intestines all this while, safely under control so long as I was reasonably healthy, has now seen fit to spring to fullest life and run wild through my system now that my immune system is busted down to nothing. The official word, I learn later, is "typhlitis." I have typhlitis. And because I'm in no condition to fight off the infection, there's a distinct possibility that I may die. My digestive system has shut down. Not merely are my intestines inflamed, the infection has created a mass of material inside, referred to by doctors as the mass or the obstruction. I can't eat, I can't shit. It's really, really painful.

Better yet, the mass (and, really, I looked like I was pregnant, I'm sorry no one thought to take pictures) is pressing my organs up against my diaphragm such that it's really difficult to take a full breath. But I'm so fucked up I don't really notice and have to have my shallow breathing pointed out to me. They get me on oxygen, one of those tubes with the umlaut-prickles for up your nostrils.

Owwwwwwwgh! You gotta make it stop, they gotta make it stop. I can't really hear them talking about infection, because all I can really focus on is the mammoth pain in my gut, the pain, the pain, give me something for the pain!

The fact is, nobody's really telling me anything. And as the pain begins to recede a bit (I think they were giving me morphine by this point, but how the hell should I know for sure), and as I try to figure what they're telling me, I can see the gap between the expressions on my doctors' faces, on my parents' faces, and the words they're telling me. I know that there is plenty that they're not telling me.

They are not leveling with me. It is worse than what they're telling me. It could be fatal, I know it for a fact. Because there is talk of surgery, an operation to get at my intestines and drain the infection that way. And I know that this is the last thing (maybe literally, heh heh) to do to a cancer patient with no immune system. An operation could kill me. So if they're talking about it then it certainly means the infection could kill me. The certainty starts beating in my head like a pulse.

This is July 3rd.

There are two alternatives. An operation, or the insertion of a "naso-gastric" tube in order to drain my intestines (also known as a stomach pumping). Somehow I have the idea that these options were presented to me as a choice.

The stomach pump. Description thereof. The entire universe went black. Entirely black except for a tiny blue pip which zigged wildly but distinctly around the lower-left quadrant of what was now my field of vision, and which I understood later was my eyeball reacting to the end of the NG tube whapping against its underside as the doctor struggled to force the tube through my sinuses. The doctor had my head down in her grip as the nostril rape continued. I dropped my cup to the floor and began to puke up everything in my stomach. The doctor let go, stepped back, freeing me, and I straightened up to see the room returned around me. The doc and I faced each other, one of us panting slightly more than the other. She still had the tube in her hand.

Doc: "Well, that's usually what happens the first time we try it." [Comedic pause]. All right, we have to try the other nostril now.

[Description of second and ultimately successful NG tube insertion attempt is omitted by order of me.]

***

*A*N HOUR LATER I WAS hooked up to the pump. I felt as if Mike Tyson had punched me in the nose and basically kept going, driving his fist through my nose and down my throat and then just basically leaving his fist where he'd gone. There was tape all over my nose, holding the tube in place. The outer end extended past my face, to a sealed pump jar on the war. Already the tube was working, filled with slowly moving goop from my belly. The obstruction. Very slow moving bloody pea soup, yum yum, slowly moving past my eye.

***

*T*HE VISION THING

Then came the hallucinations. Simple enough at first: a haze of thrashing lines in my cellphone display window, a steady manifestation crossing and recrossing the tiny screen in a fury, distracting me from reading numbers and text. I thought the phone was shorting out, dying. But soon the same thing happened to my IV unit: lightning-slashes of black cutting through the digital read-outs. I blinked, looked away, looked back, saw them still.

Later I watched similar weather settle down upon my laptop: impossible flickerings on the monitor, manic noodle contortions, impossible to get a lick of work done. I knew it was me, my brain, my eyes temporarily unable to process the particular light of electronic displays, and I was not much concerned about it; this nuisance couldn't last, and after all, the room itself, the bed and fixtures and ceiling, the fingers I waved in front of my face, all remained reliably stable. I was just a little sleep-deprived, was all I figured, and of course pumped full of satanic medicines besides, so no marvel if my vision grew a little cloudy from time to time. Surely this would pass.

It spread. Next I remember staring at the nearest wall and the lines roaming there now, faint but persistent and alive. Each wall in the room swiftly became a giant etch-a-sketch board running full-tilt, as if in time-lapse photography, doodles manipulated by some unseen hyperactive child. This became so annoying that at some point I forced myself to rise from bed and approach one of the walls, expecting the skittering patterns to vanish upon close inspection. They did not. With my nose nearly pressed to the wall's painted surface, I watched the manic geometry continue. Some boundary had been crossed.

A nurse had taped a sheet of paper to the wall across from my bed, on which she wrote down my daily blood counts, figures of far less import to me then than the dancing patterns that surrounded them.

Bugs next. Or what I took for them: boiling legions of furious specks upon the surfaces of my room, scuttling, scurrying. And not bothering to keep themselves to the corners of my eyes either, but arrogantly right out in view. The nerve!

Here came the colors. The room decided it liked to flicker and it kept this up merrily.

My brother in law came to drop off the *New York Times* early one morning. I saw him in the doorway and told him that from where I lay on the bed, he seemed to be flickering and splitting, as if on a dying picture tube. No dope, he quickly excused himself from the room. I'd have run too.

I had plenty of time to brood upon probable causes: sleep deprivation, medicine, the onset of fever. The only thing that kept my fear to a minimum, at least at first, was the knowledge that these *were* hallucinations, that they could not be real. It helped that I'd had some passing acquaintance with hallucinogens in my college years.

And all this in the broad light of day! You can imagine what my PlayForm visitors got up to at night: night was worse. The faces came, birthing out of angles and the darkest shadows. Low, flat gargoyle leers anywhere my eye turned. The bathroom was the worst, naturally the worst came from there. I never remembered to close the door, and through the aperture arms emerged, claws, glittering eyes, demons perpetually on the verge of erupting into the room. I saw these things as you see these words in front of you. Not out of the corners of my eyes but in full view.

One night the bathroom door was open far enough for me to see the mirror over the sink, to see the high coatrack/hooks and lights of the IV unit reflected in its depths, and I saw it become one of my ex-girlfriends. She'd been the most manic-depressive of them all, the one I sank into the most, the most wounded and hurt of all. I saw the form of the slowly blinking IV unit become her in the mirror in full accusation mode, silent and glaring, waiting and watching. Sometimes she was joined by others, some evil partner, who with her and was sure to do some deserved evil upon me.

Slow-motion waterfalls of molten sheets of candy: leprechaun green, Christmas red, yolk yellow, all lit from within by self-sustaining glow, never ending, flowing everywhere. The world's longest and most glorious home movie, faded Kodachrome Super-8 film—maybe some occasional 16mm from when Dad got a bonus—spliced together from every childhood weekend and summer vacation, every excursion to the movies circa 1967-72.

It was replay from the onset of my remembered consciousness, up to the dawn of puberty and the realization that life was far more hideous/complicated than I'd imagined. I hallucinated a hallucination of my childhood, a flickering magic lantern with streaks and bubbles. The Jersey shore, Lake Oscawana in New York outside Peekskill, the Atlantic City boardwalk, spectacular science fiction epics on screens forest-tall. *Fantastic Voyage, Planet of the Apes, 2001.* Always summer, always summer. Everyone is laughing. Amusement park. Cotton candy, taffy, lemonade, all of it one great sheet of a movie.

The color television in my father's parents' old house, its radioactive chromotones. Nobody ever did seem to learn how to adjust the levels on that thing. Fleshcolored actors. Overheated chemical greens, Vietnam greens. *Animal Kingdom* with Marlon Perkins, sponsored by Mutual of Omaha. An eternity of Lawrence Welk.

They settled in, established tenancy. I dreamed awake, I dreamed asleep. With open eyes in broad daylight I saw the inching colors, the lines, the bugs. The instant I closed my eyes I saw, with precisely as much clarity as if they were before me with my eyes open, natural landscapes, building interiors in succession. With my parents in the room, I calmly told them of the visions, closed my eyes and told them that I was now in someone's spacious apartment. I began to walk around in it, described out loud for the benefit of my (presumably horrified) parents the layout, the view of the window.

Lucid dreaming: I knew it was a hallucination so I had control of it...the paradox, these uncontrollable hallucinations that I was yet able to control by walking about within them and on occasion summoning up desired sights.

In the apartment I saw mail on the occupant's desk and picked it up and opened it. I pushed the dream as hard as I could, wanting to see how far it would go before dissolving, and it was only when I took a letter out from an envelope and attempted to read it aloud that the creation faltered. The letters on the page skittered like drops of spilt mercury as I attempted to focus on them. The stationery, the desk, the room in which I viewed all this, remained conspicuously solid.

I was at one point taken by stretcher to the radiology department for x-rays, for CAT scans, and I'd close my eyes and find myself in rooms of blazing neon: ceiling, floor and every wall each a single immense panel of thick colored glass within which beat horrible white strobes... the glowing gas. Horrible discos of nonstop green and red, high-lit by strange flashes of white light.

Then came the first breaths of psychosis: recurring visions, whenever I slept or napped or merely closed my eyes, of some gargantuan hotel/ casino/spa/resort, some swollen and multi-tiered adult/funland sprawl stuffed with shopping galleries, eternally ascending escalators, impossible scenes of indoor beaches under scalloped ceilings. The crucial point was how often this scenery was repeated; I saw it so frequently, on such an uninterrupted loop, and so consistently similar each time I saw it, that I became convinced it was being transmitted to me *from outside my head*, that it was only masquerading as a dream.

This was the crucial thing, that it *repeated*... so it seemed that it was an actual commercial for an actual resort being transmitted to my brain, that I had fallen victim to the most sinister subliminal advertising ploy ever yet devised. This horrible mall actually existed somewhere. This meant that also actually existing somewhere was some broadcasting station transmitting infomercials for this place. Perhaps it was just outside the hospital, perhaps it was within the very grounds of the hospital itself, broadcasting on a frequency that could only be read by cancer patients. Maybe only patients undergoing chemo and transplant like me.

Yes, folks, that's right. I stopped understanding that I was hallucinating. I thought what I saw was real. I was slipping into paranoid schizophrenia, no need to tell me that now.

I remember (or I believe I remember) ranting to a nurse about the injustice of this as I was being helped onto a stretcher for another trip to radiology. How dare the hospital allow such experimentation, were they aware that patients were being subjected to these awful synthetic dreamwaves...?

There's nothing in the hospital records about this, so either the nurse didn't bother to tell anybody or just felt sorry for me and kept my ravings to herself.

I was so angry! And once I came to this understanding about the broadcasts, I clearly sensed that employees of this advertising station were alarmed that I had figured them out. *The patient in Room 7025 is onto us! He's too clever! He's going to unveil us to the world!*

...I was on to them and their little schemes, two people as a matter of fact, and they spoke or wrote to me the name of their organization, the sinister company that was sending out these transmissions. I struggled to sit upright and reach for my notebook and pen, exerting every bit of strength remaining to me in order to write down the name of the organization, because I was going to get them. Boy, once I was out of the hospital and on my feet I was going to write about them and expose them to the world, them and their implanted dreamwaves, then we'd see who was crazy!

This was the pivotal moment, of course, when I forgot that I was hallucinating, stopped knowing I was hallucinating, when I passed out of my mind.

I cannot remember when it started...if the hallucinations came before the onset of infection, were enhanced by it, or were the vanguard of it.

Why were they taking me for x-rays? Why?

Mom: You told us there was an Indian in your room.

Judith: You called to say you were going to be in the next James Bond movie with one of the nurses.

The psychotic break : Waking from a nightmare nap which somehow included characters from *The Simpsons* (specifically Bart Simpson and Milhouse van Houten) and characters from the original *Star Trek* (chiefly Spock and his mother) and some Hitchcock-style plot involving me being falsely accused of murder. I woke convinced that I was wanted by police...intergalactic police.

My terror was real, and was only compounded by the fact that when I rose from bed, I helplessly splurted diarrhea on the floor....like a bloodstain. A severed limb. I was convinced that the very next person who walked through the door would see my shit on the floor and have all the evidence they needed to tie me to a murder (a murder had been committed, I just wasn't sure whose, only that I hadn't done it but was certain to be convicted of it).

In a panic I hid in the bathroom, appalled by the naso-gastric tube swinging from my face. This, along with my bald head and my hospital gown, may have had something to do with my impression that I was in a science fiction movie. I started looking around for a razor with some thought of using it upon myself and ending this misery. It is a very good thing that no one entered the room, because even now I don't know what I would have done if they had: screamed, confessed, begged for mercy, done harm to myself. After several minutes I began to calm down, to realize that I had been dreaming, that the dream was over and I was safe.

Chapter Sixteen

THE OBSTRUCTION

NOW THE ROOM FILLED WITH dream. I don't know what they gave me or in what quantities but I know there was morphine. Now I saw objects set not against the backdrop of the room but billowing clouds of imagery into which I entered fully. I went away and entered other places. I was an extra in the Infinite Director's Cut of the Martian version of *Gone with the Wind/Apocalypse Now.* Leering, teetering dreams. Kodachrome home movies in sickly colors, weird memories of old family trips that never occurred, childhood dinners out in restaurants long-vanished, comic book panels, rollercoaster rides, green smoke, the decks of ferry boats pitching beneath me in islanded seas, me hanging on for life. Always pushing.

I asked for ice and I got it, slowly feeding myself the chips of ice. I watched bubbles pass in the tube and I read faces in the bubbles, wise Asian men smiling under conical hats. There was a boat and the boat kept approaching turns in the river. There was always another turn, all I had to do was make it to the next turn and the next. Dawn had to come, that was part of the bargain, I knew that dawn was good.

Night was the worst. Lights out in the room, Flittermice all about, scraps of ghosts out to play. Lurkers and prowlers pushing out of the walls. Shadows that walked, breathed. Mirrors that stared. Always, always, always the fingers at the fringe of my eyesight, fingers outstretched.

No matter how you turn your head there is no way to see everything around you all at once. The boogeyman knows that, and that is where he stays. He doesn't want you to quite see him; that would spoil the fun. Ruin his reputation. After a while you stop turning your head, quit trying to catch him.

At this point there is no way to tell the precise causes of these visions. OxyContin withdrawal. Sleep deprivation. The Melphalan. The Melphalan in combination with the umpteen other medications my hospital records tell me where in my system at any given moment. Or one of those umpteen other medications in itself.

The hospital, naturally, ultimately did what they could for me: they gave me more medications. Thorazine in this case, which appears to have done the trick.

But there was something else coming over the hill, the likeliest cause of all. My hallucinations were in all probability fever dreams, because I was mounting a fever. With my immune system down to nothing, my blood levels down to what is officially called the nadir, I was getting sick. I had acquired an infection.

1950's epic style, sword and sandal Hercules deal, voice over:

In an age of scum, he was king.

He tamed the Mole People. He conquered the Rock People. He brought the Fire People to heel. And for 15 years he used them all to run a very successful family-restaurant franchise in the southern United States (shots of families enjoying mole dinners cooked over burning rocks; big neon sign out front of restaurant: Fire! Rocks! Moles! All you can eat for $3.95!)

Then he went mad, and he raised a great army of sabretooth tigers to wage war against the entire known world. Would he be victorious? Or would he end up the master of ceremonies for a new TV variety show called Hell, That's Okay!

Look, that's what I found written in my notebook. For real. I suppose you could do better in the middle of a stem-cell transplant hallucinatory state? You don't think it's funny? *Fuck* you.

THE NATURE OF THE OBSTRUCTION

He was my brother, and I ate him. I saw all the goodness and purity and sweetness in him, saw his strength and selflessness, saw the great man he would become. All the kind deeds and wonderful works, saw the family he would make, the loving wife and children, saw his attention to others, saw his limitless capacity to give. I saw he was everything I would never be. So I killed him. In the dark of our mother's womb, before anyone knew of either of us, I smothered him as he slept.

And then, to hide the evidence of my guilt, to hide forever the fact that this unspeakable act had even been committed, I ate him.

Bit by bit, morsel by soft morsel, I forced his body down my throat. I did not hurry. I had time. Less than the full nine months, true, but time enough for me to devour him in secret. He was my brother, and I ate him, but I never quite digested him or passed him out. For 44 years he remained closer than by my side—he was in my side, my little brother (which of us would have emerged first, I wonder, if I had stayed my hand from murder? Which of us would have been the little brother?), and as I grew larger and even into adulthood, he stayed lodged within my gut, hanging on and on. He was not really dead, of course, he was only sleeping.

He never bothered me in the slightest, out of the goodness of his heart, because he was so good. For 44 years he was too good to be true, but it turns out he was smarter than even I knew. He was waiting patiently through the decades for the best time to strike and take his revenge. When I was at my weakest, he did. Indeed he did. He blew himself up, my unborn twin, he spread himself through my guts and nearly blocked me to death. Or maybe he never meant to kill me, only to scare me, only to let me know which of us was boss, before allowing himself to be sucked out of my guts. That green goop snorkeled out of me backwards, up my throat and out my nose to parade past my stoned eyes and into the pump bucket.

Je vous salue, mon frere. I couldn't have done a better job myself.

This what my vision revealed to me: the true nature of the obstruction.

Chapter Seventeen

THE RECUPERATION

EVENTUALLY THE NASOGASTRIC TUBE IS clamped as a test. Clear liquids are started. Then solid foods. Then the doctor comes in and tells me the obstruction is still there—don't eat solid foods.

All the while I am thinking: what has any of this to do with cancer? What has any of this to do with my bones? Anybody would get sick if they were hauled in off the street and subjected to this treatment. How is this making me better?

But nothing bad happened. More x-rays and CAT scans. The obstruction goes away. I can eat. I spend a week with the tube unhooked from the pump but still in me, since they don't want to take it out too early then have to reinsert. Then the tube comes out. Then I feel like they're kicking me out, when the discharge comes.

NOSFERATU

IT'S DEFINITELY NOT ABOUT THE BIKE

As I rounded the last curve of the Tour de France course and bore straight into the Champs-Élysées, the sea of spectators on either side of the raceway went completely mad. French, British, Italian, German: citizens from every nation on Earth, it seemed to me, chanting my name in a deafening roar of intermingled accents. The gendarmes (that's what they call policemen over there!) could scarcely contain the surging riot. The sun shone down gloriously, my legs cycled faster into an easy blur, and the breeze of triumph made the yellow jersey on my back ripple like the American flags I saw waving in so many hands.

"USA!...USA!...Josh! Josh!...USA!" (Some smartass with Monoclonal Gammopathy of Unknown Significance shouted "MG-USA! MG-USA!")

My gorgeous wife waved to me from the observation stand beside the finish line, while next to her my tour sponsors openly masturbated into the ESPN cameras beaming the race across the globe. Ejaculating actual cash money! Gorgeous Euro-models hurled their perfect naked bodies into my path, crying out in various tones of erotic promise. As I swept across the line, I rose from my bicycle to stand proudly on the pedals at full height, lifting my fists from the handlebars and pumping them in the liberating air. Victory! Victory! Victory!

Okay, so I made that last part up. In truth, the only two-wheeled vehicle I rode in the immediate wake of my hospital stay was a wheel-chair, and not even under my own power. The nurse, wonderful Nurse A, took care of that, rolling me out of Room 7025 for the very last time (Adios! Mi casa es su casa!), then along the floor to the elevator for the seven flights down followed by the considerable push through several corridors of several hospital wings. By this time I'd already traveled farther than I had in weeks.

To the parking garage's elevator and up to its baking roof. All I did or had to do was keep my computer bag clutched safe in my lap while my older sister strode beside us with my suitcase: our little mini-parade of discharge protocol.

I'm wearing actual clothes for the first time since I was admitted (though with a daddy diaper strapped underneath my jeans, which I'm hoping I won't really need, and also hoping nobody can notice). I'm also glad that my shoes fit on my feet.

It's a busy day at the hospital that July 12, and my sister had to park her SUV all the way up on the garage roof, and it's about 90 minutes into the afternoon. In my first moment out of doors in three weeks, rising from a wheelchair on the top of a vast concrete building in the middle of a Philadelphia summer, I get the full BBQ-cookout-effect, one great swat of tropical heat falling upon my body and settling there. Maybe I *wasn't* hallucinating back in my room, maybe I really *am* living in *Apocalypse Now.*

Can't say as I'm complaining: the heat is a pleasure, the burn and humidity like strong arms over my shoulders, a welcome, a broader pulse and temperature to ponder now: the world's and not simply my own. What's that over my head? It is the sky again, whitened as desert bone in the haze. Yeah, I remember the sky. Howdy.

I get one last human hug from Nurse A. I can't believe she pushed me all the way from my room. Why, after all the things I've seen her do, all the reeking endless details I've seen her and all the other nurses and staff attend to, does that one thing seem so angelic, beyond the call of duty?

A flurry of promises to meet again under better circumstances, and then Margot and I depart. I am demobilized, a civilian.

Mid-day traffic isn't bad: everyone must be at work or on vacation... or maybe in the hospital. We're up in Bucks County soon enough. At my request, Margot pulls over at a strip-mall convenience store, so I can get out and check my bank account at the ATM inside.

There's a real thrill, muted beneath post-chemo sluggishness but real all the same, as I walk out of the van on my own and into the store. I'm the same as any other earthling, my baseball cap snug over my patchwork hair so no one's the wiser. The collection of my printed account statement, the confirmation that my last monthly paycheck was correctly auto-deposited in full, is simply the frosting on the cake. What really matters is that I'm flanked by aisles and aisles of cake, artificial-ly-flavored, -colored, -sweetened and preservative-pumped cake and cookies and doughnuts and muffins and loaves, fluorescently-lit and air-conditioned. Look at me, back in the midst of plastic candy bags and bubble-gum ultra-packs and multi-gallon soda containers swollen as the thumbs of giants. Look, there in the freezers: trough upon trough of fatty-batty ice cream! Just like before I went into the hospital! The world goes on! It's all still there!

The thought of actually eating any of this filth disgusts me. I've got no appetite, my belly still feels like it was punched in by Godzilla, but still I'm glad to see God's bounty in all its larger-than- life-size array. Life goes on! Vive le commerce de proximite!

CNN: Israel's gone into Lebanon, seeking Hezbollah hide.

My nephews are at summer day camp, and my brother-in-law's at work, so skycap service as we arrive at Le Château Grande Soeur remains my sister and me. The dogs inspect me as I settle on the front sofa, giving me the sniff-over, and I actually wonder for a moment if they'll let me pass. I've heard of dogs, not to mention other pets, reacting negatively to people who've had chemotherapy or other sorts of complicated medicinal treatments. But I seem to be accepted. The dogs can't know me too well, anyway, so what's my new smell to them? I watch Yofi with her weak hind legs drag herself tremblingly around the room, turning a corner and going out of sight. That immensely stoic animal, always contriving to move forward without any hint of complaint—and I mean *no* complaint, not canine-type nor any other sort, no growling or snapping or whining. If I ever noticed the brave dog before, that was nothing compared to how I studied her now. I could stand to learn from an expert.

For instance: this is July 12, and I haven't taken a single flight of stairs since I left my apartment on June 20...and even then I was on my way *down*. The spare room my sister has set aside for me in her house is all the way on the second floor. There must be something like 12 separate steps for me to climb in order to get up there. (Thirteen actually; I went back and counted). My sister carries my two bags up but she's not about to carry me, fireman-style or otherwise. I'm responsible for that one.

So with one hand on the nice wooden railing I set my right foot up on the first step and then the other foot on the next step, and then the right foot again up on the next higher step, and...well, I suppose if you're old enough to be reading this, you're old enough to know how to walk up a flight of stairs, so I'll conclude by saying that my first journey to the second floor was a great success, real *National Geographic* stuff, and done in such style as to promise no trouble with traveling between floors from that day forward.

The room I've been given is the computer room, across the hall from my oldest nephew. The bed's made, the curtains are drawn; I can look out across the neighboring lawns and houses, the driveways and backyard pools, the disturbingly sidewalkless avenue that runs through it all. Revolutionary Road itself.

This room is nice. Like a real room in a house! A raised wooden bed like a canopy bed without the canopy. There's an empty chest of drawers for me to put my clothes in, so no more living out of a suitcase.

I see where my brother-in-law has his computer and his high-speed internet connection, where I can plug in my laptop and go to town. My sister even tells me that the cleaning service she uses has been informed in advance that my room is off-limits for the duration. Oh boy, I feel like a big shot now.

Not sleepy but tired. The distinction must be made. Not sleepy but tired, no energy, the plug pulled.

In the corner there is a box of adult diapers that the hospital gave me to take home. Turns out I never need them. The box sits there till I dump it.

How my skin itches. My legs are constantly itching, I expect from the experience of skin swelling then subsiding from edema. My genitals feel terrible, and not in a good way. The skin down there feels constantly raw, parchment-like, not just itchy but like it will tear with the least pressure. It wakes me up at night, gets so bad I have to rub Vaseline on it because simply walking is at times too uncomfortable. It lasts a couple weeks.

So I'm getting settled domestically, and go back downstairs. The lay of the land. Here is my handle, here is my spout. I have a few things set out where I can put my hands on them quickly: my prescriptions. Those DVDs: The Simpsons, Monty Python, P J Harvey and Portishead.

There's a lot of stuff to go over. My sister and I look at the prescriptions I was given: Flagyl (an antibiotic to keep the muck tamped down in my gut), Lexapro (for depression), Clonazepam (for anxiety: wheeeee!). Also, somewhere along the way I lost my vial of Ambien; perhaps the nurses took it and kept it that night they busted me. I could get the prescription refilled, but Margot keeps dodging the subject. This is how we do things in our family. We don't say No, we don't say why we don't say No, we just don't say anything. The very idea gets the shrug-off. She does promise me a barbershop appointment for the next day, to crop my scalp once and for all.

We also check the schedule for the nurse's visits. I'm still rating house calls at this point. In two days a nurse from home health care, as directed by the hospital, is due at my sister's to take blood samples for lab tests. The mood meds I'm already on from the hospital must be doing their work, because I don't feel particularly anxious or tense about any of these upcoming tests, or even about my situation in general. I'm subdued, that's for sure, but not all that worried about the future, about those blood tests, about learning how much my transplant may or may not have taken hold.

In an inverted way, I am possibly optimistic. I feel I've been through the worst, passed through the rapids, went over the falls. I did my share of the fighting and now it's up to somebody else to hold up their end of the bargain; I've done all I can and I'm not going to worry about it. If my counts are going to stay poor, if the myeloma is going to remain, it's not for my lack of trying to fight it. I've done all I can and if I continue sick or get worse, well, it's somebody else's fault.

It's beginning to sink in how discombobulated I am. While I'm delighted to be out of the hospital and breathing the air, I'm slow. It's so good to be in a human environment, a lived-in place, but there are disconnects. My mind floats. This is what's so exasperating sometimes about being a cancer patient—or fighting any serious illness, I suspect—you can't tell what effects are being caused by what. What is a side effect and what is the disease? Which one of your treatments and medications is causing you to feel which way?

So, what is it: residual craziness? Chemo brain? (My money's on that one). The mood meds? Not to mention low blood counts, which just may have something to do with it too. Mix it all up and you get a confused customer.

I watch one *Monty Python* episode after another, and while they register in the most objective way ("Yes, this is clever,") I never laugh out loud. I know it's funny but I don't feel it. What's weird is how abstracted everything's become...as distracted and fried as my brain is, you'd imagine comedy would work directly, going straight through to my animal components, but such is not the case. *The Simpsons* likewise. I recognize the comedy but it doesn't register.

Forget reading. I can't take in two paragraphs before distraction sets in.

Forget writing.

Later my sister goes out to fill the prescriptions and to pick up her boys. I get settled on the sofa, which is something I'm going to get used to. Something else I notice: it's cold in the house. Colder than the air conditioning would seem to be responsible for. There's a blanket on the sofa that I wrap around myself. Here's something else for cancer patients to learn about: hairlessness after chemo. Body hair is fur meant to keep you warm, meant to trap your body heat, and without it you'd be surprised how cold you can get. And we haven't even shaved my head yet!

The boys are home from camp. They are running around. The house routine is manifesting itself. On comes the TV. Out come the video games. Snacks, shouts, circling dogs. "Hi, Uncle Joshua." Yeah, hi.

I don't recall setting foot out of doors once that day since I came in.

Evening, and time for my first Flagyl pill. They're almost nickel-sized, but it's not the pill that I have a problem with, it's the water. One swallow from a glass filled from the kitchen tap and I recoil like I've been given brake fluid. What is this stuff? I hold the glass up to the light, expecting to see an obvious flaw: unsightly cloudiness, particles of lead, a mouse. There is nothing of the sort: The water is as clear as my mind is not.

"What's the matter?" my sister asks.

"Oh my god, this water."

"What's the matter with it?"

"I can't drink this. It tastes like salt or something."

She sighs over her idiot kid brother. "That's only normal. Things are going to taste funny to you for a while. Didn't you notice this before? In the hospital?"

Apparently not. In the hospital I wasn't noticing much of anything, and what I did notice about food then was that I didn't particularly care to eat it. The precise taste of things wasn't an issue, and if I did notice it, I must have figured its bad metallic taste was only par for the hospital's course. I was in a hospital: food was supposed to taste like that.

But now, in a human home, in a suburban habitation, the fact that an innocent glass of water from the kitchen tap tastes like run-off from a bauxite mine is difficult to ignore. I frown at my sister.

And I am an idiot. Of course much of the literature I've read in the previous months—ever since my diagnosis—has mentioned this evident fact. Distortion in taste is bound to attend upon chemotherapy;it is something to be expected and lived with. But I am sluggish, having trouble not only adding two and two to get four. I am having trouble simply placing two and two together within the same space/time coordinates, never mind getting any type of sum as a result. All I know is this water tastes like shit.

"How long is this going to last?"

"Oy. For as long as it does. You just have to put up with it, Joshua. It's still the same water. Please drink it."

There isn't time for extensive philosophical discourse upon the subject. This isn't the sanitarium in *The Magic Mountain*. This is a house in Bucks County, suburban Philadelphia. My sister has children to pick up, groceries to purchase, arrangements to make with neighbors and colleagues that have nothing to do with me. I am extremely fortunate that she made the time to pick me up at the hospital and bring me home. Because even now that's she's gone on family leave from her job, is on a part-time schedule for the duration, she still has a great many other responsibilities.

I wonder how she manages to do it all. Why she doesn't work part-time all the time, why does she work at all, and how does she manage to hold it all together? Anyway, she has to do things around the house, (laundry, take care of the dogs) and outside of the house (pick up her two boys, shop). My job is to stay inside the house and not get infected and die. And shut up and drink the nasty water.

***

MARGOT HAS MADE AN APPOINTMENT for me at the local barber, though by this point a haircut is more like scraping snow off a windshield than a cut as such. I could probably do the honors myself but it wouldn't be a neat job.

We head out into the heat to go to the strip mall where the barber is. There is something military about all this: the heat, the ultimate cranium crop, the seen-it-all barber. Those *Apocalypse Now* referents won't go away.

Docile as a lamb. Out in the heat again I'm once more reminded how lucky I am, in terms of having someone patient enough to help me out. There's no way I could be handling this. I need somebody to help me get my haircut. In my frame of mind, I don't even care about a haircut, I'm even pleased enough that there is some hair on my head, I don't care what it looks like, that I look like a crazy person.

Thank god there's someone around who takes an interest in my appearance, who takes some familial pride in my appearance since I no longer do, and who troubles herself to make an appointment with the barber and take me there. I learn later that she had explained my tonsorial needs, being a cancer patient and everything.

So hot out. Walking slowly to the barber, who is politeness himself. This is the family barbershop in the strip mall, where my nephews go. The guy is smart enough not to make small talk; he just sets right to work. Of course, with today's styles being what they are, a chrome dome is not out of the ordinary, nothing special, par for the course. Part of the current crop, har! Everything is being taken care of. The work of a few minutes. Nice and professional. Reminder #413 that I am not unique, my situation is not anomalous, others have been this way before and society is prepared to deal with them.

So: a look in the mirror. I have to admit the head looks better.

***

NASTY TASTES ARE NOT CONFINED to water. Let us now praise nasty tastes. It's sort of a moot point, seeing as how my slugged gut is not exactly clamoring for chow. But I see that someone's been planning ahead, and the fridge is packed with all sorts of things just waiting to be taken out and heated, thawed, defrosted, microwaved.

Here is the soy milk I like. Here is some soy chocolate milk. Very thoughtful. Here is some soup in the freezer, in solid blocks of orange, vegetable-studded packets, like warped building blocks.

I am actually able to focus on the instructions, slash the packet as directed, rest it in a microwave-proof bowl and set it going for the required time and heating level. Six minutes later and I'm looking at some bubbling soup.

More fun to make than it is to eat: spooning the heated stuff into my mouth is less than exciting. Tastes like oatmeal. But the point has been made. I'm more than a little functional, can prepare food for myself, and am feeling that massive gratitude for those who have enabled me to get to this place.

I can picture myself at this moment back home, and then I can't picture it. I imagine it is just barely possible in my present condition that I could get from my apartment to the supermarket and back with some amount of groceries, but I also imagine that would be the end of it for that day. How could I possibly do anything else? I would not have the strength left to prepare the food, maybe not even to put it away in the fridge and cupboard. Right now I don't have enough energy for the basics of taking care of myself, only enough to take ultra-grateful advantage of what others have done and are doing for me.

The truth: I am dependent on others.

That first night I sleep in a regular bed. The sorry fact is that the hospital bed was more comfortable. The food may have been unsavory. There may have been staff coming in every two hours to take my vital signs. There may have been no view to speak of from my windows and nothing pleasant whatsoever. But that bed was designed to perfection. My back never hurt once. Am I fantasizing? Was it just the meds that kept me loving that bed so much? Or are those beds really so well designed that I should buy one, to hell with the cost, to hell with what it would look like in my home?

The bottom line is I can't sleep. The bottom line is, home sweet home or not, I'm not comfortable. I take the little baby doses of Oxy, but they only seem to fuzz my thoughts, not put me under. They make me too distracted to sleep. The slash of lamplight through the louvered shades. The deathless clock. The iPod with its slowly draining battery. Later I will learn what a perfect combination Ambien and the iPod make in terms of falling asleep, but that is months away.

But things are different: my body is talking. Is this illness lingering or the slow crawl back to normalcy? My skin itches terribly, though when I look there are no signs of rash. I suppose it's the swollen skin resuming its shape. It's like there's sonar inside of me, pinging and sounding.... the light through the suburban window. Lots of time to think, too much time to think, but as well the inability to hold a thought. Brainwaves all over the map.

One thing for sure, though. Television is still too boring to watch. One afternoon I sit with my nephews as they watch some kiddie channel on cable, some nonsense early-teen epic about unpopular girls and nerdy guys trying to get into some party, some girls trying to sneak out to a hot party or get into some great nightclub blah blah...I can't take it. At one point, my oldest nephew says, Here comes my favorite part.

Your favorite part? I say. You mean you've seen this before?

Yeah?

How many times?

I dunno. A shrug. Five or six.

Who am I to be critical? How many times did I watch *The Monster* or *Frankenstein Meets the Wolf-Man* when Channel 29 used to run those five times a week on Monster Chiller Horror Theater? Still, this teen movie blows. What my nephews were interested in: my catheter. Say hello to my little friend. How I flush out my catheter. This gets their attention. Does it hurt? No, I don't feel anything.

***

*T*IME FOR A WALK....THROUGH THE suburbs. The heat. My rambling thoughts. The ease of getting lost. Almost never seeing anyone at all, let alone on foot. Possible to walk for several minutes without seeing anyone. No sidewalks. If I see anyone at all they are on the immediate grounds of their house, fixing up or puttering on the lawn. Of course you see no one walking: there is no place to walk to. No squares, no parks, no coffeehouses, nothing but the curvilinear plots of houses divided by streets with Dutch names. There are no sidewalks, there is nothing to encourage walking. Not that I get dirty looks or anything like that....

I discover something wonderful about my sister and her husband. They have a coffee maker that they set up on the kitchen counter before they go to bed, with a timer that kicks in around dawn. So when even I, sleepless Sam, slip downstairs in the early of morning, there's a pot already brewed. I guess I'm backwards—what do I know aside from my laptop and iPod?—but I'm pretty amazed by this thing. Oh what a sucker I've been all these years, brewing my coffee in the mornings, actually standing there and waiting for it to brew, when I could have had a machine do it for me overnight!

Anyway, "I am glad for the gourd," as Jonah said, glad for the coffee hot and available, glad the whole thing's been taken out of my hands, glad I don't have to fumble-finger through the process of making a cup every morning, waking everyone up and, in my zoned-out mindframe, botching the whole process. There's a pot of coffee waiting for me every morning! (Well, not all for me, some for my sister and brother-in-law too).

Best of all is the regularity of it. I still want my morning cup! I still need my morning cup! Blessed routine. I am learning: it is out of these unassuming processes that our lives are made, our little rituals. The rosary counts of the secular. "My life has been measured out in coffee spoons"—as if this were a bad thing.

***

*T*HE DAY OF THE REMOVAL of the catheter comes in late July. It really is shameful how lousy a journalist I was then. Anyway: how they did it. The removal was in the same radiology department where I had the damn thing put in in the first place. So I'd had two months living with it, which in retrospect doesn't seem like much.

There is a nurse with her blues and her clear plastic visor, like a welder's mask. I really regret not asking to keep the catheter. Lance Armstrong says he kept his. I should have thought of it.

The big thing is it's my first day out on my own. Margot gives me a ride to the Neshaminy Falls rail stop, and I wait for the train into town. There's a stop right in University City, a short walk to the hospital.

Then I get out and take a cab ride to my house. What fun! It's so good to be home!

Have I ever been away from home so long at such a short distance? No I have not.

To be home alone! Is there a greater pleasure? No there is not.

I sit there in the heat for a while. That's what I remember doing, nothing else. Just sitting there. There was even the temptation to phone my sister and ask her to please bring my things down, to just stay. I don't know why I didn't. I must have known I wasn't finished recuperating yet. That I needed more time in the kiln. That I didn't have the strength to be on my own yet.

Somehow I got it together to get back to the train station, ride the rails back to the rugged frontiers of Bucks County. I have no memory of doing this.

Chapter Eighteen

THE END

ONE MORNING I WAKE UP to something new, something so old it's new: an appetite. I actually feel like eating something.

For THE END: "Unfortunately, I remain alive. Very sorry about that. Or at least still alive as of this writing, this moment, this sentence. I'm afraid this will undercut the point I've been trying to make about the seriousness of myeloma. How bad can it be, you understandably ask, if this character is still alive to talk about it. Some cancer. Now, my father/mother/daughter/uncle had an operation, had their xxxxx removed, had chemo and all and still died of cancer. Now *that* was cancer, so what is this fellow moping about? So, by having the poor taste to remain alive, am I actually doing the cause of myeloma research a disservice? Shouldn't I do the polite thing and die, maybe die right now (cough gurgle rrrrrrrrrrhghgggggggggghhhhhh) just to show you all how nasty this can really be?

But what'll I do for an encore?

I am often reminded of that great 1937 screen comedy, *Nothing Sacred*. That'd be a good name for a cancer memoir, by the way... or in the case of a myeloma patient with collapsed lower vertebrae, *Nothing Sacral*. The great Carole Lombard plays a young woman in a small deadly dull town right out of (rather too obviously out of) Sinclair Lewis who is mistakenly given a terminal diagnosis. A New York City newspaper decides to sponsor her last days on earth, really show her a good time Manhattan style—screwball comedy style, at the cost of the exclusive rights to her story of course, and she's a big hit, the plucky kid. New York just rolls over for her, parades, fireworks, everything free, everything the city of New York has to offer given to her free and clear, because she's such a brave and beautiful kid and she's going to die in a matter of months, weeks, days... Everyone who sees her bursts into tears, falls in love with her and her bravery and surrenders to her heart and soul and bursts into tears.

Then, of course, that diagnosis was a mistake, and the weeks go by and the weeks go by and Carole Lombard doesn't die. People (they are New Yorkers, after all) start to get a little impatient, and then a lot impatient, and they start wondering why she doesn't even look sick and when the hell is she going to die already?

I won't tell you the end because I don't want to spoil the ending for you. But I will say that the beautiful and talented Carole Lombard died at age 33, by the way, when her plane flew into a mountain. And *Nothing Sacred* was remade as *Living It Up* in 1954 with Martin and Lewis. Also as *Imminent Death Syndrome* from Mr Show.

But I can't help being reminded of the story. As if I'm asking for your pity and then your continued pity and then some more pity on top of that. It's not like I came back and won the Tour de France or anything. I just got, for the moment, and as of this moment, better.

But nobody with myeloma gets *better* better. They just get better for a while. And then we lean into the other curve. Which is that *no*body gets better better. Everybody dies. Everybody. What makes this particular story of any distinction? And if I die, am I just another shmuck/statistic who died of cancer? Why is this cancer different from all other cancers? What up, my knotty headed myeliggas? With your back bones operating on hair triggas? A word to my myeliggas. (Just a frustrated comedian? Sexually frustrated, to be sure).

Of course, at some point in time, I will be dead, quite possibly of some cause other than myeloma, and that may even be so far in future that many of you reading me now (now = 2007) will be dead too. So—assuming this book remains in print long enough, which isn't fucking likely—to my very future, possibly as yet at this moment unborn readers, I address myself to you: Hello, I have cancer. Had, had, had cancer, a form of cancer called myeloma.

I say had because now I am dead. Even if I had survived the cancer I am now definitely sure to be dead. Of something. So to you I say: once I was alive, even as you are now. But now I am dead.

To which you might surely reply: So fucking what, grampa? And turn back to your ZVD or neuro-implant pornshow or whatever it is you jerks of the future are diverting yourselves with. Yes, ha ha, everyone now living as I write this, will, in 100 years, be dead. With a few exceptions. Jerks. Die hards, if you will.

You see how we're all in this together. You non-canceroids will not escape, you're no better off than myself than by a few years, minutes really by the geologic records, seconds actually, tick tock—ask not for whom the bell tolls and all that.

It's that terrible terrible shock when you hear that you or someone you love is diagnosed with cancer or some other serious disease. It's the raising of that pesky mortality issue. And for those who hear about cancer (just to restrict this to cancer), I think this is the terrible thing, the reminder. It's why people back away. It's why you're scared to tell people when you get the diagnosis, because you see them backing away, you see the horror, the shock, the grief. You feel like something in a horror movie, the monster out of the closet, and you die just that little bit more inside.

It's not like, well, if I can avoid cancer, then I won't die. Everybody dies. Everybody. It's as though this is any consolation, but you know, if it wasn't myeloma, it would have been something else. Everybody dies.

Because nobody deserves to crawl around in a deteriorating body. (Well, mostly nobody). Because if you can cure this, we'll have improved the quality of life for so many people. People will live a little longer, and they'll be happier, and the quality of life will improve for everyone they know. I'm not sure people should live forever, but what are you going to do, roll over and die?

Why did I write this? Why, to publicize myeloma, of course. If not to inspire then to slightly educate. Life is so extraordinary that I find even its mutations, *especially* its mutations, to be worthy of close scrutiny. To raise awareness, as they say in the literature, as they say in the literature of all diseases, all cancers, all charities, to raise public awareness—so that's what I'm trying to do here. Between your newspaper and your morning show and your favorite online sites and your reality shows and that latest YouTube video, here is another form of cancer you've never heard of and this is it. Let me tell you about it, it's really quite interesting; pull up an x-ray and sit down while I tell you.

Lance Armstrong: "I didn't beat cancer. The doctors beat cancer. The drugs beat cancer." I like that he said that.

I am getting nostalgic for the early days of my cancer diagnosis and treatment. Missing the Fox Chase Cancer Center. The cat who moved, who I took in, who huddled shivering in his litter box because it was the only familiar thing. If anything demonstrates how sickening, how mentally ill, nostalgia can be, this is it.

I have entered the time of anniversaries. I have made it. One year post-diagnosis, two years post diagnosis. I remember when.

Nosferatu and Sanjuro. Two movie characters, solitary figures who stalk the screen, with their own peculiar rules of conduct, and whose presence inevitably leads to the loss of blood. Sound like anyone we know?

L'Avventura and L'Eclipse. Fata Morgana and Lessons of Darkness. Army of Shadows. (Eclipse, Shadows, Darkness...what is going on?)

***

I'M DISCHARGED FROM THE HOSPITAL for good. This is it. The paperwork was all filled out. Not that I remember signing my name to any of it, but here the pink copies are, in my files, before me on my desk. I don't feel like a "cancer patient" or like someone suffering from "multiple myeloma"—in fact, my back feels great. I feel like some displaced person... the cancer has gone out of my mind and what it is is that I've recovered from is the hospital stay itself. That I've recovered or am recovering from not myeloma but the treatment for myeloma.

This is so unfair, so viciously unfair to the people who saved my life. There's the horrible temptation to blame everything on them, on the doctors, on the treatment, on the tests. To think: if it wasn't for the doctors, I'd never have learned I had cancer. It is all their fault. They poke me and siphon my blood and make me piss into a jug I have to keep in my fridge, and in return they tell me horrible news.

This is one of the worst things about being ill, I've found. Or that I've found out about myself: that I'm full of untethered hate and anger ready to direct itself at the nearest target. This target just happens to be the people who have uncovered my problem and are working to save my life. The people who did and do save my life.

Later I will watch *La Notte,* its opening scene of some terminal patient, treated with morphine, visited by Mastriaonni and Moreau. His hospital room in Milan, the view to the cold alienating city outside, the traffic. He doesn't look that sick to me. Can't help thinking of *The Hospital,* and the woman I dated briefly a decade and a half ago who told me how turned on she got by the quasi-rape scene.

The seventh floor. The bulletin board of cards. Thank yous. A heartbreaking handwritten note, shaky because it is a hand unused to writing, an uneducated hand, or because it is itself a hand diseased and/or aged, and/or otherwise infirm and/or stricken with grief.

It is not right, it will never in a million years be right, that this woman should've had to scribble *my life will never be the same without my daughter…* What kind of a world is this where a mother has to write a letter like that? And what kind of world where a mother finds she *can* write a letter like that?

I turn my head; I cannot bear it.

THE END

Chapter Nineteen

EPILOGUE: LIGHT THE NIGHT

START WITH THE IMAGE OF the balloons in the dark. The rain, the onset of evening. Then flashback....

Sometime late in August, I notice a brochure at the front of my local bagel shop: spokesperson Cindy Crawford, on behalf of the Leukemia & Lymphoma Society, is promoting Light the Night Walks throughout the United States. These Walks, like so many others for so many terrible diseases, are intended to raise awareness of, and money for, blood cancers. The brochure is commendably organized; is, in fact, from the Eastern Pennsylvania Chapter of the L&LS, and lists the six separate Walks scheduled throughout the Philadelphia area over the coming autumn. The one in Philadelphia proper is on September 30th, along the Delaware River downtown waterfront, the strip known as Penns Landing. Cindy Crawford, eh? Turns out her brother died of leukemia.

Penns Landing. That's just a modest walk from where I live. And the Capital-W Walk is on a Saturday night, when, let's face it, I won't be doing anything in particular. Okay, I'm going to become an activist.

The brochure tells how to register online for the Walk with the L&LS, at which point you're given access to a webpage you can personally customize, and to which you can direct people for online contributions. Their software is pretty good. It's just a matter of minutes before I've got the page up and running on the L&LS server, complete with a self-posted snap of me crossing the famous pedestrian crossing at Abbey Road, London, in 2004, as made famous by The Beatles. It's a picture of me walking, get it? They let you set a personal fundraising goal, which you can track with one of those rising-thermometer graphs. I do a little thinking: if I can get 20 people to contribute $25, I'll get $500. Yes, it's possible! I even create my own snappy headline: *Help Me Walk Blood Cancers Into The Ground.* That'll get the money pouring in....

Oddly, it does. No sooner have I e-mailed the URL to family and friends than e-mails begin turning up in my e-mail box, auto-alerts about donations: you have received a donation from.... And another. And another. In less than a week I've got my five hundred dollars. So I do the unthinkable. I raise the amount.

Frankly, I hardly have to do any of the work. My younger sister e-mails I don't know how many of her friends, and donations start pouring in from names I don't know. My sister demands a list of donors (I can get it online) to compare with her list so she can shake down whomever hasn't contributed yet. My mom steps to the plate. A thousand dollars, fifteen hundred.... Perhaps I'm in the wrong business.

There are Rhoads staff on hand. Some of them I don't recognize, some seem familiar but I can't remember their names. Others, who nursed me through the infection and obstruction, telling me I was sicker than I had supposed, sicker than family had let on. "We were worried about you."

I tell them I hereby repudiate anything I said while raving.

Now I'm at the bowl of the Grand Plaza where, months before, I had danced in the sun. There are bands onstage, some free snacks. Rain comes on, then leaves, blowing off by sundown leaving the air fresher, better-smelling. There are balloons, the red outnumbering the white by what appears to be 20:1. The lights come on, their electric candle light ("her name was Lola"). First the light is steady, then it flickers. The L&LS has spent a lot of money on these things. The rain, the cold.

The bunched masses of balloons in the wind.

I've got too much junk in my backpack: an umbrella, a weighty flashlight, a swag of shirts. Why do I do this? WHAT HAVE I GOT IN THIS THING?

My hip joints are killing me. I shouldn't have been standing for so long. I slip a couple of short-acting OxyContins out (I'll feel them later) and look at the streams of balloons.

No one's ever said this, but I presume the intent is to replicate the look of a healthy bloodstream: the strong red cells coursing along full of oxygen, the occasional white balloon cell as sentinel. Though I can't help remembering *Fantastic Voyage* and the scene where the white blood cell swallows up the bad guy. I was five years old. I was scared. I wanted to scream as much as the actor.

***

*A*ND SUDDENLY WE'RE MOVING, GOING north alongside the river instead of south, the direction opposite to which I'd been facing. Past the battleships in dock. They've set it up so nobody has to cross any busy streets, least of all Delaware Avenue/Columbus Boulevard , but I worry that we're the only ones seeing ourselves, that we're not getting the message out. What must the few people think who see us along the riverfront, or briefly passing the intersection of Front and Chestnut? How do they read the red balloons, whose lettering can't truly be made out in the dark? Do they think this is an early manifestation of Halloween? Just another AIDS awareness walk by pesky faggots? Just another Take Back the Night protest by just some more nagging dykes?

I fear the healthy bloodstream imagery is lost on the general public. I see precisely one camera from one local news station, and later there's no media coverage: no TV, no radio, no print.

But there are these fundraising walks and runs and bikeathons every weekend. This is the thing, this is the maddening thing. How are you to make people notice the particulars of a single illness, of a single ill person? I certainly never gave it much thought myself until I got cancer. Well, what can you do? Here I am, hundreds of pages after I started talking about myeloma and I'm still not convinced anyone not connected to the disease gives a damn. Do you give a damn, reader? I don't blame you if you don't, I'm sure you have other troubles of your own. But thanks for making it this far.

There are signs put up along the route by the L&LS, lawn-signs along the side of the walk route, a little like the Burma-Shave. Some are informative little snippets about the group and its funding: "Last year the L&LS raised....." Some are exhortations to us walkers: Every step you take brings us closer to a cure. Some are statistically clinical: *Leukemia is the main cause of death of children under 20.*

Slightly more than halfway through the walk I come upon one of those as it relates to myself:

The survival rate for myeloma is still only 32.4 percent today, making it the most difficult blood cancer to treat successfully.

I take a picture of the sign, just for the record books, and then I do the only thing to be done: I continue walking.

Chapter Twenty

AFTERLIFE

MARCH 25, 2007: A TRIP to Anguilla (rhymes with vanilla) following my first official remission on last week of December. I book the trip the first week of January, and a good thing, too, as rooms are at a premium the week I plan to go. And it all works out, and I enjoy everything. Even the slight slips: the delay leaving the Philadelphia airport, the one connection missed, the piece of luggage misplaced. Those things just don't bother me, and all is easily resolved.

I get the high sign from the doctor the last week of December: all clear. Full remission. The excitement is tempered somewhat by the diagnosis being dependent on a bone marrow biopsy, and the realization that I'll be getting one of those every year for the rest of my life. (So, maybe there won't be many after all).

Remember how I used to fantasize about the tropical beach early in 2006, back when I was being depth-charged by Thalidomide? The white sand, the blue water, the constant sun. An alcoholic beverage in my hand. That's what I wanted, and that's what I booked. Somewhere I read that the Caribbean's best beaches were in Anguilla, so that's where I went. Second half of March, 2007. Expensive, exclusive, low-key Anguilla.

Which is how I happened to be on St. Martin one overcast Sunday afternoon. Like something out of Vonnegut, St. Martin is the French side of St. Martin/St. Maarten, a single island and especially popular tourist destination in the Caribbean West Indies, an island divided between a French side and a Dutch side. Reputedly the smallest single land mass on earth shared by two governments (they haven't seen my parents' house). So small is the island that you can get a fair look at both sides in the space of one day, riding the local bus route that connects the respective capitals, Marigot and Phillipsburg.

St. Martin/St. Maarten is a 30-minute ferry ride from Anguilla—you can easily see the islands from each other so I thought that Sunday I'd really live it up, do some island hopping, check out the French highlife. What I didn't know was that Sunday afternoon was naptime in Marigot, more or less, and while I was able to find some lunch, there wasn't much else to do. I toured the ruins of the colonial fort, I looked at the harbor, I looked back at Anguilla. The sky was coming over cloudy and there wasn't a real sense of excitement in the air.

What better time to tour the cemetery?

That's right. I've heard there's a bus that can take you around to the Dutch side, but before I make it over there, I want to check out the long narrow cemetery by the harborside. It rates a mention in my Lonely Planet guide, so maybe there's somebody famous buried in there. Memories of the cemetery in Montparnasse flood my head. I oughta be able to get some good pictures. There's a cement wall that I can peep over, and it does seem a little picturesque in there, like a New Orleans cemetery: flat tomb markers, wild vegetation, bottles, notes.

I walk around the wall till I find the open gate. As I stroll into the grounds, an old fellow in thin old clothes is coming out, and as we pass each other he mumbles something in a language I don't know. He has his hand extended toward me, making a sort of grabbing gesture, turning his hand from one side to the other, muttering all the while. He has a voice so low I assume it's French or some related dialect. Everybody has their hand out. No, I'm not giving you money, sir, no.

I proceed in and it's not bad, this cemetery, everything gray and lots of overgrowth. Am I morbid? Or just an explorer? I want to see what an old cemetery on the French side of a Caribbean island looks like. With an authentic old guy poking around. Local color. No markers, no indications of any famous dead. The site is long and narrow, in order to fit into the geography of the harbor. There are some markers with fairly recent dates, some brief lifespans, lives cut short. Engraved sentiments, embedded photos. I wonder about Anguilla: I haven't noticed any cemeteries on that tiny island (though that would conclusively prove my insanity, wouldn't it, if I spent my Carribbean vacation sniffing out graves? Like I'm doing now?), and the ground is so rocky. Do they bury their dead at sea? Makes sense.

I have company: a rooster stalks the graves. Local color. Some well fertilized growth here for him. Where are his hens? Does he live here or, like me, is he just paying a visit? Rust-orange body, full black tail, proud red comb. He keeps his distance from me, but not in a rushed or hurried way, as I follow him for a while, snapping my pictures. Tough customer, literally not letting his feathers be ruffled. Maybe somebody he knows is buried here.

Only he may have the pleasure of my company for a while longer. It turns out that the cemetery is a bit bigger than I thought, or sound is muted under the overcast island sky, or that old fellow knows how to maneuver quietly. When I get back to the gate I have a nice little surprise: it's locked. The metal-barred gate is closed and padlocked. I look at it, incredulous.

Revenge of the caretaker! Pretty funny, I have to admit. Now I re-member his outheld hand, the turning motion he made over and over: pantomime of locking. And of course he was talking to me, telling me he was going to close up.

So this is how I come to be locked alone inside a Caribbean cem-etery on an overcast Sunday afternoon. Not the worst way for a fellow to choose to end a book such as this. A man could get into the spirit of this, and the joke of it sinks in pretty quickly—even if, especially if, that old fellow did this deliberately. Adventure in the Caribbean. Real boy's adventure book stuff: locked within the old French colonial boneyard. This is what I came here for.

But I don't stay. Escape is easy. Without moving from the gate I spot a single cinderblock leaning against the wall. The wall itself is only head height in any case, so I step atop the block and hoist myself up, swinging my legs over the wall, dangling for a moment on the other side. It's only about a foot and a half drop, and I hang there just long enough to understand that I could never have done this a year ago. An eighteen-inch drop would have killed me, the thought of it paralyzing me with fright, but now here I am, clambering over walls and out of graveyards. Progress. True story.

And for the time being, I leave the cemetery behind.

Goodbye, ladies and gentlemen. *Au revoir* for the French side. Nice seeing you. I'll be back eventually, one of these days, sooner or later, for a longer stay, for certain. We all will, all us living together. But just not today. Cross my heart and hope to, anyway.

Chapter Twenty-One

THE SISTERS SPEAK III

MARGOT

Joshua enjoyed a three-year remission from the initial transplant. After those three years, treatments, side effects and life with multiple myeloma resumed and continued for the next 7-8 years.

Joshua's oncologist had originally planned for him to have tandem transplants (two autologous transplants) 6 to 12 months apart. Because of the potentially life-threatening complication he had of neutropenic enterocolitis, or typhlitis, plans for the second SCT were out of the question. In fact, Joshua refused his oncologist's requests for years to have a second SCT because of the serious complication he'd suffered. It was only years later, when the myeloma had "gone wild" and a last ditch, "hail Mary" pass was needed in attempt to control the disease that Joshua relented and agreed to have the second SCT.

JUDITH: The Colostomy

It was the week of Thanksgiving 2009 when Joshua called Margot and me. He was having extreme abdominal pain, had started vomiting, and told us he was taking a cab to the ER. Since Joshua hated the idea of being in a hospital, I knew it had to be bad if he was taking himself there.

We got to the ER shortly after he arrived. Despite Joshua telling the ER doctor that he felt like his bowels were blocked, it seemed the doctor's opinion was that this was a routine case of the flu or pneumonia, and a chest x-ray was ordered. When Joshua's belly started swelling up like a watermelon and he began vomiting large amounts of watery green fluids, the ER doctor's demeanor changed. The surgeon on call was consulted, examined Joshua, and looked at his chest x-ray where she could see free air where there shouldn't be up under his diaphragm. This was a sign of a bowel rupture/perforation, and Joshua was taken for emergency surgery, basically having his life saved by this astute woman. The bowel perforation was a complication from Joshua's many years of prolonged steroid use beginning when he was diagnosed (thankyouverymuch, multiple myeloma).

Hours later, prior to seeing Joshua in the recovery unit, we were told the surgery was successful but Joshua would have a temporary colostomy for a few months. Also, instead of surgically closing his abdomen and trapping any bile or digestive contents that may have escaped during his bowel perforation (creating another life-threatening situation), the surgical site was left open for any remaining drainage and would heal on its own. By the time we saw Joshua, he knew he had a colostomy in the abstract, but it didn't register with him what it really meant.

That revelation hit as the grogginess disappeared over the hours. Although Joshua was grateful to be alive, he was repulsed when he understood that his large intestine had been surgically rerouted, sutured and an incision made in his abdomen so his feces would leave his body through a surgically created hole—and be collected in a bag.

It took him days before he'd look at his abdomen, but it helped him in a small way when he was told it was temporary. His hospital stay was blessedly uneventful and his surgeon was pleased to arrange discharge on Thanksgiving Day, with recuperation at my house. A hospital discharge earlier than expected sounded fantastic in theory, but on a major holiday it meant a closed hospital pharmacy. A closed hospital pharmacy meant no prescribed pain meds in a nice white paper bag to tote home with you.

Things stepped into high gear with my husband, who worked at the hospital, collecting Joshua and setting out in search of those precious pain pills. They drove to and called every chain pharmacy in our area with increasing panic. The chain stores, one by one, simply did not have the needed meds in stock.

When my husband and Joshua arrived at my house where our small extended family already was, I found myself apologizing to him for the table full of food that he had no appetite to eat or the desire to accept how it was going to exit. His head was swimming from everything. What are you thankful for on Thanksgiving, Joshua? Why, my sister's little neighborhood non-chain pharmacy that beat out all the chain stores by coming through with the prescribed pain meds.

Joshua's recuperation at our place was a tough adjustment period for him. In addition to dealing with a colostomy that wasn't disappearing anytime soon, he also had the open wound that I needed to clean and dress daily. Besides knowing that Joshua loved his privacy, I was very sensitive to the fact that he was embarrassed, overwhelmed with his medical situation, and feeling a loss of dignity. "Let's talk about how to shower with your wound. Let's talk about your colostomy in regard to what you're eating." Keeping Joshua's dignity became a forever high priority for me, a personal theme that the myeloma would force us to revisit periodically through the years.

Early one morning, the colostomy bag's adhesive fittings (onto the body) became loose while he slept, and his feces leaked onto the bed. We learned together how the adhesive fittings were only good for about five days. Thankfully this coincided nicely with the visit by the Colostomy Guru, as we dubbed the nurse who kindly and sensitively talked to Joshua to try to help calm him while explaining colostomy care.

Joshua was mortified by the Colostomy Bag Accident, which was exacerbated by having to change out the packing material on his 3" long by 2" deep wound daily. We couldn't simply put a nice clean bandage over it—instead it required my pulling out the long strip of gauze full of drainage, like a bad magician's trick, and repacking the wound full of clean gauze with the help of a hospital-grade stick.

Joshua and I learned to coordinate our timing so he could take a pain pill prior, leaving enough time for its benefits to kick in before I started. Those first few days we'd give each other a pep talk before I took off the bandage because after the first night I told him he couldn't ask me again, "Do you really know what you're doing?"

Before the visiting nurse came the first time (the Monday after Thanksgiving, which seemed like forever since the surgery), Joshua and I began fretting that the wound didn't look right. He had to use a mirror to see it, and to both of us it was looking more disgusting. But when the nurse showed up, he explained that all that specific type of disgustingness meant the healing process was beginning from the inside out right on time. Who knew!

As Joshua found his rhythm, he looked to return home as soon as possible. He was cautiously getting the hang of the colostomy and he took over his own wound care since he knew that was his ticket back to his own place. We got him back to his home with lots of food, and I'd continue to take him to his scheduled follow up appointments with his surgeon. She felt it was safest to wait 6-7 months before reversing the colostomy, so later in the summer, Joshua underwent successful surgery. I'd be remiss not to mention that as the surgery date drew nearer, during a pool party at our house that summer, Joshua got a kick out of covering his colostomy by casually wearing his scuba diving suit.

*J*UDITH: The Second Stem Cell Transplant

Joshua's 2015/2016 year-in-review included too many hospitalizations and health concerns. His myeloma was becoming more and more aggressive as it pushed back against the various treatments. Joshua dealt with pneumonia plus an added bonus of *Clostridium difficile* diarrhea, often called C. diff. He had increasing calcium levels leading to hallucinations, intensifying nosebleeds, and a visible lump on his head where the myeloma was obliterating his skull and replacing the bone with its own vile matter. The skull bumps became an external disease monitor: we could actually see as the myeloma was growing. The high M-spike levels led to mild kidney failure, and he had horrific back pain, rib pain, shoulder pain, pain and pain.

Joshua accepted his doctor's advice to try a second stem cell transplant the end of May in 2016. Compared to his physical self, years earlier at his initial transplant, this version of Joshua was resigned, frightened due to the first transplant's complications, and physically frailer.

The extras following Joshua's second transplant included nausea, massive swelling in his legs making it extremely difficult to walk—much less wear shoes—and a nasty return of C. diff which sent him back into the hospital for a week. He had to use supplemental oxygen temporarily, and was unbelievably exhausted. Those complications, and a hefty supply of new medications (not to be confused with his current medications which were already quite hefty), came along with Joshua when he was discharged late June and began Operation Stem Cell Transplant Recovery 2016 at our home. Joshua's recuperation was slow and grueling; he would stay with us into August.

Joshua was my brother but also a patient. I was his sister but also a caregiver. The massive amounts of medications Joshua came home with were all put into an Excel spreadsheet by my husband, listing drug names, doses, days and times of when to administer. Joshua continued to use this list until hospice care nearly a year later.

The practical portions of the day included coordinating a circus-like varying schedule of the visiting nurse, physical therapist, infusion nurse who took the blood for workup, the driver who picked up and transported the blood, and the procedures we did ourselves. He received a 2-hour magnesium IV drip that we had to learn to hook up ourselves—no fun, but we got the hang of it, no pun intended. There was also daily catheter flushing, walking around for the edema but also rest the legs and—oh, visits to his oncologist. Factor in that Joshua could barely get out of bed due to his massive exhaustion which would plague him for weeks. He would later say that he couldn't remember much of this initial time. I'm not surprised, due to how much his body had been through and his lethargy. Although the exhaustion would decrease, it was something he would deal with for months to follow.

After the first month with us, Joshua's health came round a little more and more. A sense of normalcy (or new normalcy) returned as he was interested in meals, increased his interaction with my kids, became interested in his mail (both snail and "e"), and wanted to sit outside. Let me take this opportunity to mention that no matter what was going on with Joshua in his life, he always took the time to ask those around him how they were. The private man who asked about others. This period of time was no different and I will always remember and value that beautiful aspect about him. The physical signs of healing were the bulge in his head receding (myeloma matter disappearing) as well as what Joshua and I came to think of as Car Ride Sensitivity.

Car Ride Sensitivity was how careful I had to drive to avoid every pothole, take all curves slowly and coast on uneven portions of road so he wouldn't become unbalanced and yell from back pain. The day I drove him back to my house from the hospital after the stem cell transplant as well as to his oncologist two weeks later: Code Red Level High Car Ride Sensitivity. It was like I was oh-so-carefully driving an unbuckled Ming Dynasty vase.

However, weeks later during a drive to his oncologist I accidentally hit a pothole. I tensed, my apology nearly out of my mouth as I snuck a side look at Joshua who was relaxed and comfortable while staring out the window. I told him what happened and we marveled that some major myeloma beat-down must be at play, which it was. The stem cell transplant had successfully lowered myeloma's M-spike to 0.7. That was fantastic news and gave Joshua "breathing room" (his words, not mine) while his oncologist tried out new treatments and combination new/old standard treatments in the coming months. Unfortunately, the partial remission was short-lived. In October the myeloma began to simmer and gather steam, growing again despite the treatments and hitting its full stride by December.

MARGOT

The couple years before Joshua's death were a near constant battle against the multiple myeloma. Joshua blew through one failed treatment after another. Oftentimes though, "failing" a standard treatment is the only way to become "eligible" for a clinical trial. In addition to being "eligible," one must have a good performance status (PS). This means being up and about more than half the day and not having any active or uncontrolled issues like an infection or wildly abnormal lab values. It was getting harder to say Joshua had a "good" PS. Imagine a boxing match where the same boxer keeps losing every round but somehow gathers the strength for the next round. The myeloma kept progressing and winning. Now he'd even developed 2-3 masses, or lumps of myeloma, on his bald head and breastbone that were external measurements of his cancer. These lumps would enlarge to peach size or regress depending on whether a treatment had failed or if he'd gotten a (short-lived) positive response. With all the pain, toxicity and symptoms he endured then, I kept waiting for him to say *Stop, I'm done, that's enough*. But he kept going.

Joshua agreed to salvage chemotherapy, a three- or four- drug infusion combo cocktail that was a last-ditch effort to see if his numbers could get good enough to get into the CAR-T cell clinical trial where a spot was being held for him. This is a type of immunotherapy, where the patient's own T cells are drawn from the blood and infected with a gene for a chimeric antigen receptor (this is the CAR part). This gene causes the T cells to target any cells that express a protein called CD19, which is found on tumor cells of several types of blood cancer. It is called immunotherapy because the immune system is being reprogrammed to specifically fight the cancer.

To be eligible for the study, patients had to be off any treatment for a month before the T cells were drawn. Joshua had the salvage chemotherapy, was discharged from the hospital and then had a scheduled oncology office appointment about a week later.

I knew about the appointment, but was surprised when he called me from the emergency room late in the afternoon that day. He'd been sent there by his nurse practitioner because he had a fever and was neutropenic. The neutropenia was to be expected a week after chemotherapy, but neutropenic fever is always bad news, so sending patients to the ER is standard operating procedure. The ER can draw blood cultures to check for infection and start broad-spectrum IV antibiotics ASAP. This was pretty routine, and so was being in the ER waiting hours for a hospital bed to become available, so we were in touch by phone a few times into the evening hours while he waited for a bed.

Sometime close to 10 pm I got called by an ER doctor to tell me that Joshua had developed problems breathing, and that it was bad enough that they'd wanted to put him on the ventilator. He refused. Many years prior, Joshua had completed his advanced directives and made himself a Do Not Resuscitate (DNR), meaning no breathing tube, no chest compressions, and no electric shock. They had him on a BiPap oxygen mask, which was the most they could do while respecting his wishes.

I got to the hospital in record time and ran from the parking garage into the ER entrance, slowing briefly as I passed the security guard at the metal detector. I was directed to one of the corner rooms and could see my brother, his entire face surrounded by a heavy clear mask. Imagine a baseball catcher's mask of heavy clear plastic. What I could also see was Joshua's entire chest rising up and down so fast, non-stop, as he labored to breathe. The mask fogged up in sync to his rapid chest heaving.

Before I could get to his bedside I was approached by one of the doctors, who told me that his blood pressure had dropped in the short time since they'd called me and they'd needed to start an IV drip of Levophed (norepinepherine) to maintain a normal blood pressure. They thought he had acute respiratory distress syndrome and that he was going into septic shock from a hidden lung infection.

Since I'd worked for many years in critical care in my nursing past, I didn't really need to listen to the doctor's explanations. I knew that his oncologist calling in to talk with my sister and me now, about 1:00 am, was "the phone call to the family": the *I'm letting you know, that I know that Joshua's not going to survive this* phone call. I handed the phone to my sister.

It was the first time I thought my brother was going to die. He was suffocating. He was working exhaustedly and his chest was heaving up and down about fifty times a minute. Joshua could shake his head yes or no, but couldn't talk with the facemask on and couldn't breathe with it off, even for a few seconds. His eyes stayed closed, opening them only if someone spoke to him.

I asked him to reconsider having the ventilator support—if only for a short time, a couple days at most, to ease the workload of breathing, to make him more comfortable while trying to get the lung infection under control. He shook his head no. He was holding to his advance directives. I knew that if he became too lethargic or unconscious and could not make his own medical decisions then I could do so, since I was his medical decision-maker when he was unable. It was painful watching him struggle and so I was prepared to have him be angry with me. I knew that it was possible for things to improve, but not without ventilator support.

My sister and I stayed with Joshua and followed him as he was transferred up to the Medical Intensive Care Unit (MICU) a couple hours later. We stayed at his bedside for some time and then, slowly, Joshua began to become more alert. Miraculously his breathing eased a bit. He pushed himself onto his elbows and waved at us both to come closer to the bed. He took off the facemask and then reached out with both of his hands to grab a hold of each of ours and said "I thought I was going to die."

We were so happy to hear him speak those words. We were relieved that despite him not surrendering his DNR wishes, his breathing continued to improve and he was able to share his fear.

The miracle continued the next day when Joshua's heart went briefly into a lethal rhythm called ventricular tachycardia. This is when the heart spontaneously starts pumping so fast that the ventricles can't fill up with enough blood to pump out to the body. Normally this is a "code blue" heart shocking event, but because he was a DNR he got a bolus dose of Lidocaine with an infusion started. Within one very long minute his heart rhythm returned to normal.

Within a week or so of those events and after some post ICU psychosis and confusion, Joshua was well enough to be discharged home. It was truly a miracle that Joshua was ever able to walk out of the hospital from his final hospital stay. We were grateful he was able to get home. He was never able to receive the CAR-T cell treatment.

**March 30, 2017 by Joshua Roberts (final post)

The longer I take to post updates, the more there is to report. Unfortunately, the great majority of that is bad news. Pembro and Pomalyst have not proved to be a winning combination, nor does the current replacement (as of early March): Velcade/Nelfinovir (aka Viracept)/Dex (40 mg/week). Velcade did do me some good a couple years ago, but now even teamed up with other meds, it seems to have lost its efficacy. My numbers are out of control: IGG is 7550 mg/dL, and M-spike is 7.1 g/dL. That's pretty deadly. I'm creaky, slow, and prone to nosebleeds, and my activities outside the house are more or less limited to grocery shopping, the occasional movie, and medical appointments. My oncologist is clearly thinking that I cannot maintain the present course of treatment, and that I should seriously consider a clinical trial that would engineer my T-cells to more aggressively combat the myeloma cells clogging up my bloodstream. The trial is complicated with a tricky schedule, it could make me much sicker before any perceived improvement, but I don't have too many options left at this point. I had been hoping to travel at the end of April, just a quick trip to an island for a change of scenery, but that's been shelved for the time being. Some days (especially recuperating from the dreaded weekly "dex crash"), I can't get off the sofa.

AFTERWORD

RYING TO ADD OR OFFER a small part in closure for my brother's memoir is an intimidating task. He eloquently and openly chronicled his personal battle against multiple myeloma over the span of twelve years. His last blog entry was in March, and in April 2017 his steep decline began. Because the cancer was out of control he suffered through the worst toxicities and complications myeloma has to offer in his last months of life.

Since his death, I've had the opportunity to go through his writings, books, letters and notes he had on everything from his "to do" list, house repairs list, daily notes, travel notes, thoughts and feelings. My brother's most valued possession was the written word. Whether it be in all the letters he kept, his writings and notes, published or not, or in his valued personal book collection. It was in his notes, diaries and this *Marrow Me* memoir, that everything was "let out." As long as Joshua wasn't hospitalized you'd never hear him complain about pain, medication effects or the cruelty of his multiple myeloma. But in writing, everything was expressed. The pain, the profound fatigue, the reality of the disease and thoughts of ending it all on his own terms. I wish he'd shared more of his feelings with those around him, including my sister and me and with his circle of friends. My grief is not just for Joshua's death, but for all the thoughts, hopes and desires of his that died along the way those twelve years.

In Joshua's last couple of months the myeloma was particularly cruel. He entered hospice care on May 18, 2017. With my husband's help and support, Joshua was able to stay at our home for most of that time. I kept waiting for the typical end stages of hypercalcemia and kidney failure to occur so he could just become more and more lethargic in his confusion and "go peacefully." That's what's supposed to happen! Instead, he remained pleasantly confused with hallucinations and some not so pleasant delirium. He then progressed to agitation ... the exact opposite of what was supposed to happen. He couldn't even catch a break and experience any of the cancer's typical end of life benefits.

Joshua died on June 15th and according to his wishes, his cremains were scattered at Shark Wall Dive off of New Providence Island, Bahamas; the spot he had loved and enjoyed for scuba diving.

May we all find some comfort and peace in reading Joshua's writing. His humor, wit, purpose and soul are exposed and are missed terribly.

—Margot Roberts Sweed

REFERENCES AND RESOURCES

General and historical references

1. Hoogstraten, B., Sheehe, P.R., Cuttner, J., Cooper, T., Kyle, R.A., Oberfield, R.A., Townsend, S.R., Harley, J.B., Hayes, D.M., Costa, G. & Holland, J.F. Melphalan in multiple myeloma. Blood 30, 74-83 (1967). http://www.ncbi.nlm.nih.gov/pubmed/6028709

2. Durie, B.G. & Salmon, S.E. A clinical staging system for multiple myeloma. Correlation of measured myeloma cell mass with presenting clinical features, response to treatment, and survival. Cancer 36, 842-854 (1975). http://www.ncbi.nlm.nih.gov/pubmed/1182674

3. Kyle, R.A. Multiple myeloma: how did it begin? Mayo Clinic proceedings 69, 680-683 (1994). http://www.ncbi.nlm.nih.gov/pubmed/8015334

4. Kyle, R.A. Multiple myeloma: an odyssey of discovery. British journal of haematology 111, 1035-1044 (2000). http://www.ncbi.nlm.nih.gov/pubmed/11167737

5. Kyle, R.A. & Rajkumar, S.V. Therapeutic application of thalidomide in multiple myeloma. Seminars in oncology 28, 583-587 (2001). http://www.ncbi.nlm.nih.gov/pubmed/11740813

6. Kyle, R.A. & Rajkumar, S.V. Multiple myeloma. The New England journal of medicine 351, 1860-1873 (2004). http://www.ncbi.nlm.nih.gov/pubmed/15509819

7. Greipp, P.R., San Miguel, J., Durie, B.G., Crowley, J.J., Barlogie, B., Blade, J., Boccadoro, M., Child, J.A., Avet-Loiseau, H., Kyle, R.A., Lahuerta, J.J., Ludwig, H., Morgan, G., Powles, R., Shimizu, K., Shustik, C., Sonneveld, P., Tosi, P., Turesson, I. & Westin, J. International staging system for multiple myeloma. Journal of clinical oncology : official

journal of the American Society of Clinical Oncology 23, 3412-3420 (2005). http://www.ncbi.nlm.nih.gov/pubmed/15809451

8. Kyle, R.A. Five decades of therapy for multiple myeloma: a paradigm for therapeutic models. Leukemia 19, 910-912 (2005). http://www.ncbi.nlm.nih.gov/pubmed/15800669

9. Alberts, B., Wilson, J.H. & Hunt, T. Molecular biology of the cell, Table of contents only http://www.loc.gov/catdir/toc/ecip0710/2007005476.html, Edn. 5th. (Garland Science, New York; 2008).

10. Kyle, R.A. & Rajkumar, S.V. Criteria for diagnosis, staging, risk stratification and response assessment of multiple myeloma. Leukemia 23, 3-9 (2009). http://www.ncbi.nlm.nih.gov/pubmed/18971951

11. Kyle, R.A. & Steensma, D.P. History of multiple myeloma. Recent results in cancer research. Fortschritte der Krebsforschung. Progres dans les recherches sur le cancer 183, 3-23 (2011). http://www.ncbi.nlm.nih.gov/pubmed/21509678

Current research

1. Holstein, S.A., Richardson, P.G., Laubach, J.P. & McCarthy, P.L. Management of relapsed multiple myeloma after autologous stem cell transplant. Biology of blood and marrow transplantation : journal of the American Society for Blood and Marrow Transplantation 21, 793-798 (2015). http://www.ncbi.nlm.nih.gov/pubmed/25652690

2. Kazandjian, D. & Landgren, O. A look backward and forward in the regulatory and treatment history of multiple myeloma: Approval of novel-novel agents, new drug development, and longer patient survival. Seminars in oncology 43, 682-689 (2016). http://www.ncbi.nlm.nih.gov/pubmed/28061986

3. Filonzi, G., Mancuso, K., Zamagni, E., Nanni, C., Spinnato, P., Cavo, M., Fanti, S., Salizzoni, E. & Bazzocchi, A. A Comparison of Different Staging Systems for Multiple Myeloma: Can the MRI Pattern Play a Prognostic Role? AJR. American journal of roentgenology 209, 152-158 (2017). http://www.ncbi.nlm.nih.gov/pubmed/28418695

4. Abonour, R., Wagner, L., Durie, B.G.M., Jagannath, S., Narang, M., Terebelo, H.R., Gasparetto, C.J., Toomey, K., Hardin, J.W., Kitali,

A., Gibson, C.J., Srinivasan, S., Swern, A.S. & Rifkin, R.M. Impact of post-transplantation maintenance therapy on health-related quality of life in patients with multiple myeloma: data from the Connect(R) MM Registry. Annals of hematology 97, 2425-2436 (2018). http://www.ncbi.nlm.nih.gov/pubmed/30056582

5.   Bringhen, S., Offidani, M., Palmieri, S., Pisani, F., Rizzi, R., Spada, S., Evangelista, A., Di Renzo, N., Musto, P., Marcatti, M., Vallone, R., Storti, S., Bernardini, A., Centurioni, R., Aitini, E., Palmas, A., Annibali, O., Angelucci, E., Ferrando, P., Baraldi, A., Rocco, S., Andriani, A., Siniscalchi, A., De Stefano, V., Meneghini, V., Palumbo, A., Grammatico, S., Boccadoro, M. & Larocca, A. Early mortality in myeloma patients treated with first-generation novel agents thalidomide, lenalidomide, bortezomib at diagnosis: A pooled analysis. Critical reviews in oncology/hematology 130, 27-35 (2018). http://www.ncbi.nlm.nih.gov/pubmed/30196909

6.   Dimopoulos, M.A. & Kastritis, E. Thalidomide for myeloma: still here? The Lancet. Haematology 5, e439-e440 (2018). http://www.ncbi.nlm.nih.gov/pubmed/30290901

7.   Gonsalves, W.I., Buadi, F.K., Ailawadhi, S., Bergsagel, P.L., Chanan Khan, A.A., Dingli, D., Dispenzieri, A., Fonseca, R., Hayman, S.R., Kapoor, P., Kourelis, T.V., Lacy, M.Q., Larsen, J.T., Muchtar, E., Reeder, C.B., Sher, T., Stewart, A.K., Warsame, R., Go, R.S., Kyle, R.A., Leung, N., Lin, Y., Lust, J.A., Russell, S.J., Zeldenrust, S.R., Fonder, A.L., Hwa, Y.L., Hobbs, M.A., Mayo, A.A., Hogan, W.J., Rajkumar, S.V., Kumar, S.K., Gertz, M.A. & Roy, V. Utilization of hematopoietic stem cell transplantation for the treatment of multiple myeloma: a Mayo Stratification of Myeloma and Risk-Adapted Therapy (mSMART) consensus statement. Bone marrow transplantation 10.1038/s41409-018-0264-8 (2018). http://www.ncbi.nlm.nih.gov/pubmed/29988062

8.   Khattry, N., Laskar, S., Sengar, M., Rangarajan, V., Shet, T., Subramanian, P.G., Epari, S., Bagal, B., Goda, J.S., Agarwal, A., Jain, H., Tembhare, P., Patkar, N., Khanna, N., Punatar, S., Gokarn, A., Shetty, D., Jain, H., Bonda, A., Gota, V., Hasan, S., Kode, J., Dutt, S., Kulkarni, S., Shetty, N., Sable, N., Deodhar, J., Jadhav, S., Pawaskar, P., Mathew, L., Menon, H., Nair, R., Kannan, S., Chiplunkar, S. & Gujral, S. Long term clinical outcomes of adult hematolymphoid

malignancies treated at Tata Memorial Hospital: An institutional audit. Indian journal of cancer 55, 9-15 (2018). http://www.ncbi.nlm.nih.gov/pubmed/30147087

9.   Mahajan, S., Tandon, N. & Kumar, S. The evolution of stem-cell transplantation in multiple myeloma. Therapeutic advances in hematology 9, 123-133 (2018). http://www.ncbi.nlm.nih.gov/pubmed/29713445

10.   Royle, K.L., Gregory, W.M., Cairns, D.A., Bell, S.E., Cook, G., Owen, R.G., Drayson, M.T., Davies, F.E., Jackson, G.H., Morgan, G.J. & Child, J.A. Quality of life during and following sequential treatment of previously untreated patients with multiple myeloma: findings of the Medical Research Council Myeloma IX randomised study. British journal of haematology 182, 816-829 (2018). http://www.ncbi.nlm.nih.gov/pubmed/29984830

Resources for Patients and Caregivers

Multiple Myeloma Research Foundation
https://themmrf.org/
A patient-founded organization dedicated to finding a cure for MM. Includes links to clinics and other resources.

International Myeloma Foundation
https://www.myeloma.org
The first and largest foundation dedicated entirely to multiple myeloma.

Leukemia & Lymphoma Society
http://www.lls.org/
Support for all blood cancers.

Life with Multiple Myeloma
https://www.lifewithmultiplemyeloma.org/
On-line support group for patients.

Made in the USA
Columbia, SC
09 April 2020

91388978R00098